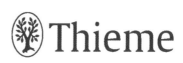

Sinonasal Complications of Dental Disease and Treatment

Prevention–Diagnosis–Management

Giovanni Felisati, MD
Professor and Head, Unit of Otorhinolaryngology
Director, Department of Head and Neck Surgery
Department of Health Sciences
San Paolo Hospital
University of Milan
Milan, Italy

Matteo Chiapasco, MD
Professor and Head, Unit of Oral Surgery
Department of Health Sciences
San Paolo Hospital
University of Milan
Milan, Italy

302 illustrations

Thieme
Stuttgart • New York • Delhi • Rio de Janeiro

Library of Congress Cataloging-in-Publication Data is available from the publisher.

© 2016 by Georg Thieme Verlag KG

Thieme Publishers Stuttgart
Rüdigerstrasse 14, 70469 Stuttgart, Germany
+49 [0]711 8931 421, customerservice@thieme.de

Thieme Publishers New York
333 Seventh Avenue, New York, NY 10001 USA
+1 800 782 3488, customerservice@thieme.com

Thieme Publishers Delhi
A-12, Second Floor, Sector-2, Noida-201301
Uttar Pradesh, India
+91 120 45 566 00, customerservice@thieme.in

Thieme Publishers Rio, Thieme Publicações Ltda.
Edifício Rodolpho de Paoli, 25º andar
Av. Nilo Peçanha, 50 – Sala 2508
Rio de Janeiro 20020-906 Brasil
+55 21 3172-2297 / +55 21 3172-1896

Cover design: Thieme Publishing Group
Typesetting by DiTech Process Solutions

Printed in Germany by Aprinta GmbH, Wemding 5 4 3 2 1

ISBN 978-3-13-199701-2

Also available as an e-book:
eISBN 978-3-13-199711-1

Important note: Medicine is an ever-changing science undergoing continual development. Research and clinical experience are continually expanding our knowledge, in particular our knowledge of proper treatment and drug therapy. Insofar as this book mentions any dosage or application, readers may rest assured that the authors, editors, and publishers have made every effort to ensure that such references are in accordance with **the state of knowledge at the time of production of the book.**

Nevertheless, this does not involve, imply, or express any guarantee or responsibility on the part of the publishers in respect to any dosage instructions and forms of applications stated in the book. **Every user is requested to examine carefully** the manufacturers' leaflets accompanying each drug and to check, if necessary in consultation with a physician or specialist, whether the dosage schedules mentioned therein or the contraindications stated by the manufacturers differ from the statements made in the present book. Such examination is particularly important with drugs that are either rarely used or have been newly released on the market. Every dosage schedule or every form of application used is entirely at the user's own risk and responsibility. The authors and publishers request every user to report to the publishers any discrepancies or inaccuracies noticed. If errors in this work are found after publication, errata will be posted at www.thieme.com on the product description page.

Some of the product names, patents, and registered designs referred to in this book are in fact registered trademarks or proprietary names even though specific reference to this fact is not always made in the text. Therefore, the appearance of a name without designation as proprietary is not to be construed as a representation by the publisher that it is in the public domain.

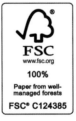

Contents

7. ENT Contraindications to Maxillary Sinus Grafting Prior To or In Association with Oral Implant Placement 128

Giovanni Felisati, Alberto Maria Saibene, Matteo Chiapasco, Sara Torretta, Lorenzo Pignataro

Videos

Foreword

This book stems directly from a long-lasting and solid collaboration between various medical specialists involved in the management of sinonasal complications of dental disease and treatment. Authors and coauthors, despite practicing in different hospitals and universities, have been working closely, sharing clinical experience, and treating and discussing patients together since the early 2000s.

The two editors, Giovanni Felisati and Matteo Chiapasco, have published in international journals several fundamental contributions to the understanding of this complex set of clinical problems spanning different areas of clinical and surgical expertise. The authors have taken advantage of their unique experience to give birth to an original textbook, drawing a much-needed map of a territory previously uncharted by the specialist literature.

In this book, otolaryngologists, maxillofacial surgeons, oral surgeons, dentists, and forensic dentists will find practical answers to diagnostic and therapeutic dilemmas posed by sinonasal complications, which frequently require multidisciplinary expertise that goes way beyond the usual study program for each of these specialties.

Such a multidisciplinary approach to patients has been the key to successfully treating the astonishing 360-plus case series presented, including patients surgically treated for sinonasal complications of dental disease and treatment ranging from fungus balls to oroantral fistulae and, again, from peri-implant osteitis with sinusitis to failed maxillary sinus augmentation procedures.

Thieme Publishers have strongly supported the book, allowing the inclusion of a large number of illustrations and offering a web-based collection of high-quality case videos. These will help readers put into practice the approaches conceived by the authors through a keen and meticulous multidisciplinary study of patients, coupled with a focused evaluation of treatment procedures and a follow-up-driven constant re-evaluation of patients.

Roberto Brusati, MD
Professor and Head, Regional Centre
for Cleft Lip and Palate
Department of Health Sciences
San Paolo Hospital
University of Milan
Milan, Italy

Paolo Castelnuovo, MD
Professor and Head, Unit of Otorhinolaryngology
Director, Department of Surgical Specialties
Azienda Ospedaliero-Universitaria, Ospedale di Circolo
di Varese
University of Insubria
Varese, Italy

Preface

From mid 1980s, important technological innovations have revolutionized rhinology and oral surgery, with the introduction of endoscopic approaches to the sinuses, new dental treatment techniques, and advanced implantology procedures. These surgical procedures have experienced major advances in complexity and extent, but at the same time related complications have grown in number and severity. Such complications, starting from the maxillary sinus, may spread secondarily to all the other nasal and paranasal cavities.

Very often, the treatment of such pathosis is performed independently either by oral and maxillofacial surgeons or by otolaryngologists, but frequently with less than ideal outcomes, a significant relapse rate, and exhaustingly prolonged diagnostic and treatment times for patients.

A transnasal endoscopic approach alone, for instance, is not able to remove the etiological factor (an infected tooth or an infected implant penetrating into the maxillary sinus). An intraoral approach, on the contrary, is not able to control the maxillary sinus ostium and other involved paranasal sinuses, restoring their drainage when required. A real multidisciplinary approach can therefore facilitate a pivotal breakthrough.

Sinonasal Complications of Dental Disease and Treatment is intended to provide otolaryngologists, maxillofacial surgeons, oral surgeons, and dentists with a practical guide focusing on rational, multidisciplinary approaches to treat these pathoses.

Readers will find a straightforward guide to rational diagnosis and management of these often complex cases through protocols that have been thoroughly validated by dentists, maxillofacial/oral surgeons, and rhinological surgeons.

Precise and concise medical protocols are provided for timely treatment of complications. When medical therapy fails, the role of functional endoscopic sinus surgery (FESS), intraoral approaches, or a combination of intraoral approaches and FESS will be specifically and thoroughly described.

Furthermore, we have included a chapter focused on the prevention of sinonasal complications following implant-related reconstructive procedures. The chapter will give precise information on how to identify and treat possible contraindications to maxillary sinus grafting procedures, such as anatomical variations impeding ventilation of the sinusal ostium.

Finally, in order to further clarify our treatment concepts, the book includes access to many surgical videos wherein we present complete clinical cases. These informative videos will be available on the Thieme website.

Giovanni Felisati, MD
Matteo Chiapasco, MD

Acknowledgments

The authors would like to thank all coauthors for the wonderful work done while writing this textbook. Everyone has made a substantial effort to create a shared vision concerning the diagnosis and treatment modalities of odontogenic sinusitis, summarizing the otolaryngological, maxillofacial and stomatological points of view. Such common ground was unimaginable only a year ago.

Special thanks go to Dr. Alberto Maria Saibene, whose contribution went well beyond his involvement in writing some of the chapters. He has had a fundamental role in preparing the photographic and video material and tying together the different chapters, and he has been our keen and focused liaison with Thieme and all coauthors.

Our sincere thanks go to Thieme staff for the kind help they have provided. This is especially true for Ms. Nidhi Chopra, Thieme Project Manager for this book, who managed to guide us through the maze of deadlines and changes to the book with the utmost patience and professionalism.

Finally, the authors would like to thank all the surgeons working at the Otolaryngology Unit, Maxillofacial Surgery Unit, and Oral Surgery Unit of the San Paolo Hospital, University of Milan, Italy, who took part in many of the procedures depicted in the book and helped create this ever-growing corpus of knowledge related to odontogenic sinusitis.

Contributors

Federico Biglioli, MD
Professor and Head, Unit of Maxillofacial Surgery
Department of Health Sciences
San Paolo Hospital
University of Milan
Milan, Italy

Teresa Bini, MD
Staff Physician, Unit of Infectious Diseases
Department of Health Sciences
San Paolo Hospital
University of Milan
Milan, Italy

Andrea Borghesi, MD
Assistant Professor, Unit of Radiology
Spedali Civili di Brescia
University of Brescia
Brescia, Italy

Roberto Borloni, MD
Staff Physician, Unit of Otorhinolaryngology
Department of Health Sciences
San Paolo Hospital
University of Milan
Milan, Italy

Matteo Chiapasco, MD
Professor and Head, Unit of Oral Surgery
Department of Health Sciences
San Paolo Hospital
University of Milan
Milan, Italy

Lorenzo Drago, PhD
Head, Clinical-Chemistry and Microbiology Lab
Department of Biomedical Sciences for Health
IRCCS Galeazzi Institute
University of Milan
Milan, Italy

Giovanni Felisati, MD
Professor and Head, Unit of Otorhinolaryngology
Director, Department of Head and Neck Surgery
Department of Health Sciences
San Paolo Hospital
University of Milan
Milan, Italy

Aldo Bruno Giannì, MD
Professor and Head, Maxillo-Facial and Dental Unit
Department of Clinical Sciences and Community
  Health
Fondazione IRCCS Ca' Granda, Ospedale Maggiore
  Policlinico
University of Milan
Milan, Italy

Riccardo Lenzi, MD
Staff Physician, Division of Otorhinolaryngology
"S.s. Giacomo e Cristoforo" General Hospital
ASL 1 Massa Carrara
Massa, Italy

Paolo Lozza, MD
Staff Physician, Unit of Otorhinolaryngology
Department of Health Sciences
San Paolo Hospital
University of Milan
Milan, Italy

Alberto Maccari, MD
Head, Unit of Laryngology
Department of Health Sciences
San Paolo Hospital
University of Milan
Milan, Italy

Roberto Maroldi, MD
Professor and Head, Unit of Radiology
Spedali Civili di Brescia
University of Brescia
Brescia, Italy

Antonella D'Arminio Monforte, MD
Professor and Head, Unit of Infectious Diseases
Department of Health Sciences
San Paolo Hospital
University of Milan
Milan, Italy

Lorenzo Pignataro, MD
Professor and Head, Department of Otolaryngology
Department of Clinical Sciences and Community
  Health
Fondazione IRCCS Ca' Granda, Ospedale Maggiore
  Policlinico
University of Milan
Milan, Italy

Carlotta Pipolo, MD
Assistant Professor, Unit of Otorhinolaryngology
Department of Health Sciences
San Paolo Hospital
University of Milan
Milan, Italy

Pierpaolo Racco, DDS
Adjunct Professor, Maxillo-Facial and Dental Unit
Department of Clinical Sciences and Community
  Health
Fondazione IRCCS Ca' Granda, Ospedale Maggiore
  Policlinico
University of Milan
Milan, Italy

Alberto Maria Saibene, MD, MA
Resident, Unit of Otorhinolaryngology
Department of Health Sciences
San Paolo Hospital
University of Milan
Milan, Italy

Alberto Scotti, MD
Staff Physician, Unit of Otorhinolaryngology
Department of Health Sciences
San Paolo Hospital
University of Milan
Milan, Italy

Sara Torretta, MD, PhD
Researcher, Department of Otolaryngology
Department of Clinical Sciences and Community
  Health
Fondazione IRCCS Ca' Granda, Ospedale Maggiore
  Policlinico
University of Milan
Milan, Italy

Alessandro Vinciguerra
Intern, Unit of Otorhinolaryngology
Department of Health Sciences
San Paolo Hospital
University of Milan
Milan, Italy

Marco Zaniboni, DDS
Private Practice
Milan, Italy

About the Authors

Giovanni Felisati, otolaryngologist, is the head of the Head and Neck Department of the San Paolo Hospital, Milan, Italy, and is a faculty member of the School of Medicine of the University of Milan. A renowned rhinologist, with more than 60 peer reviewed publications ranging from pediatric otolaryngology to skull base surgery, he has devoted much of his recent work to interdisciplinary management of odontogenic sinusitis.

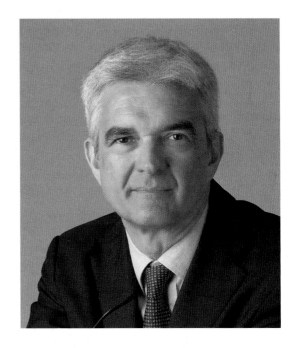

Matteo Chiapasco, oral and maxillofacial surgeon, is the head of the Oral Surgery Unit of the San Paolo Hospital, Milan, Italy, and is a faculty member of the School of Dentistry of the University of Milan and the Loma Linda University (California, US). With 250 peer reviewed publications and 10 textbook, he is a prominent surgeon and international lecturer on maxillofacial surgery topics such as orthognathic surgery and advanced preprosthetic surgery.

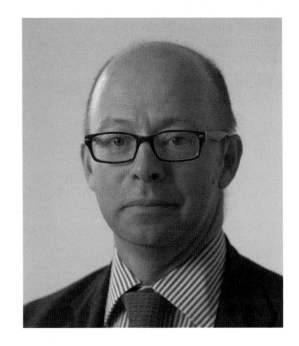

Chapter 1

Anatomy, Physiology, and Pathophysiology of the Paranasal Sinuses

1

1 Anatomy, Physiology, and Pathophysiology of the Paranasal Sinuses

Riccardo Lenzi, Alessandro Vinciguerra, Alberto Maccari, Carlotta Pipolo

Contents Overview

This chapter will focus on the anatomy and physiology of the sinonasal tract. A surgically oriented description of the maxillary sinus and lateral nasal wall is provided, followed by an endoscopic perspective. Finally, the reader will find a discussion of the physiological functions of the sinuses and the pathophysiological implications of sinonasal ventilation, with particular focus on odontogenic conditions.

1.1 Maxilla and Maxillary Sinus

1.1.1 Topographic Anatomy

The maxillary sinus is usually the largest of the paranasal sinuses. The sinus is a large pyramidal cavity within the body of the maxilla; its lateral apex may extend to the zygomatic process or into the zygomatic bone.[1] Its limits are: the orbital floor superiorly; the hard palate, alveolus, and dental portion of the maxilla inferiorly; the zygomatic process laterally; a thin plate of bone separating the cavity from the infratemporal and pterygopalatine fossae posteriorly; and the uncinate process, fontanelles, and inferior turbinate medially[2] (▶ Fig. 1.1 and ▶ Fig. 1.2). Its average dimensions in adults are: height 33 mm, width 23 mm, anteroposterior 34 mm; the average volume is 15 mL.[1]

In adults, the floor of the maxillary sinus is 3 to 5 mm below the level of the nasal cavity, whereas in children the floor of the sinus is above or at the level of the nasal cavity.

The ostium of the maxillary sinus lies on the highest part of the medial wall of the sinus and opens into the posterior half of the ethmoidal infundibulum, not directly into the nasal cavity. It is oriented slightly offset from the parasagittal plane, facing posteriorly, and is usually around 5 mm in diameter.[3] Accessory maxillary sinus ostia occur in approximately 10% of the population and are located in the posterior fontanelle area.[4]

Exploration of the whole maxillary sinus through the natural ostium (even after surgical enlargement and with angled endoscopes) is generally not possible. In particular, two recesses, more or less pneumatized, are difficult to visualize: these are the prelacrimal recess, located anteriorly to the nasolacrimal duct (▶ Fig. 1.3), and the alveolar recess, representing the pneumatization of the alveolar process. The posterior and superior walls are usually clearly visible.

Two prominences may be present on the posterior wall of the maxillary sinus. The first runs anteriorly from the upper part of the posterior wall of the maxillary sinus to the inferior orbit and corresponds to the infraorbital nerve, leaving a ridge or groove along the roof of the sinus, while the other is located on the middle part of the posterior wall and corresponds to the maxillary artery.[5]

Ridges and septa can be found on the interior surface of the maxillary sinus, and larger ones may impede proper drainage of mucus. Occasionally, a complete septum divides the sinus into two compartments. One compartment may drain into the other or by an accessory ostium

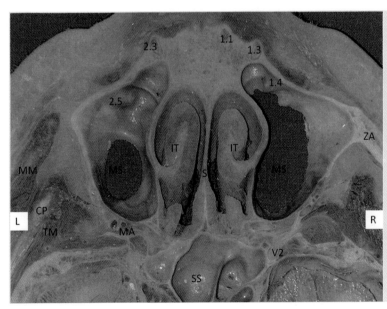

Fig. 1.1 Axial section of a cadaver head passing through the maxillary sinus (MS), seen from above. The relationship with the surrounding structures and teeth (1.1, 1.3, 1.4, 2.3, 2.5) is clearly visible. Posteriorly to the left MS, the maxillary artery (MA) is visible within the pterygopalatine fossa. CP, coronoid process of the mandible; IT, inferior turbinate; MM, masseter muscle; S, nasal septum; SS, sphenoid sinus; TM, temporalis muscle; V2, second branch of the trigeminal nerve; ZA, zygomatic arch.

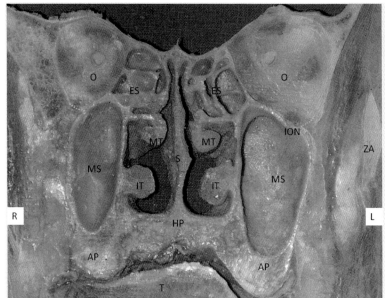

Fig. 1.2 Coronal section of a cadaver head passing through the maxillary sinus (MS), seen from anterior. It is possible to see the orbit (O) separated from the MS by a thin layer of bone, containing the infraorbital nerve (ION), and the inferior orbital fissure (*yellow dotted line*), via which the orbital contents are continuous with the infratemporal and pterygopalatine fossae. AP, alveolar process; ES, ethmoid sinus; HP, hard palate; IT, inferior turbinate; MT, middle turbinate; S, nasal septum; T, tongue; ZA, zygomatic arch.

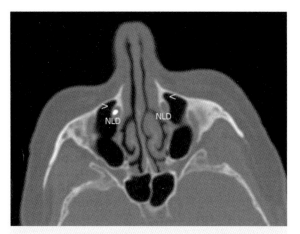

Fig. 1.3 Axial CT scan showing a bilateral prelacrimal recess (*white arrowheads*) anterior to the nasolacrimal ducts (NLD).

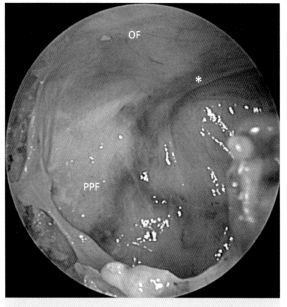

Fig. 1.4 Endoscopic endonasal exploration with a 45° endoscope of the left maxillary sinus (of a cadaver head) after wide middle meatal antrostomy. The superior wall (OF, orbital floor) of the maxillary sinus, with the infraorbital bundle partially dehiscent (*white asterisk*) is clearly visible. The posterior wall, covering the pterygopalatine fossa (PPF), can also be seen.

into the nasal cavity.[1] Ridges rising to distinct septa are called Underwood's septa and challenge the oral surgeon performing maxillary sinus lift, as they facilitate the rupture of the thin membrane during the elevation of the maxillary sinus mucosa.[6]

Other points at risk of injury during surgical procedures are the infraorbital nerves and vessels in the superior wall of the sinus and the anterior and posterior superior alveolar nerves that may be dehiscent inside the sinus (▶ Fig. 1.4).

The maxillary sinus is lined with mucoperiosteum, also called *Schneider's membrane*. On histological examination the mucoperiosteum is a double-layer membrane consisting of ciliated columnar epithelium on the inner side and periosteum on the outer side.

Anatomical Relationship between the Maxillary Sinus and the Teeth

The anatomical relationship between the maxillary sinus and the teeth is highly variable, since it depends on the pneumatization of the alveolar process. Usually the molars are separated from the sinus by a layer of compact bone, but sometimes this layer can be thin or absent, providing a direct route for odontogenic infections to spread into the sinus (▶ Fig. 1.5). The maxillary third molars have the most constant relationship to the maxillary sinus. The canine tooth or the first and second molars occasionally reach into the sinus.[1]

Innervation and Blood Supply

Nerves

Sensory innervation of the maxillary sinus mucosa mainly originates from the infraorbital nerve and its main proximal branches, namely the posterior superior alveolar, the middle superior alveolar, and the anterior superior alveolar nerves.[1] The anterior superior alveolar nerve branches from the infraorbital nerve during its course within the infraorbital canal and runs on the anterior wall of the maxilla toward the pyriform fossa, before branching and forming the superior dental plexus located in the alveolar process of the maxilla.[7] The course of this nerve has a variable pattern, and injuries to its fibers are responsible for the neurological complications of canine fossa puncture (dental and facial numbness, tingling, and pain).

Secretomotor fibers from the facial nerve originate in the nervus intermedius, synapse at the pterygopalatine ganglion, and are carried to the sinus mucosa with the trigeminal sensory branches.[8]

Arteries

Blood supply to the maxillary sinus mucosa is provided by branches of the maxillary (i.e., posterior superior alveolar artery), infraorbital (i.e., anterior superior alveolar arteries), and sphenopalatine arteries (entering the sinus through the semilunar hiatus or the nasal fontanelles).[9] An important arterial branch is the alveolar antral artery, which is an anastomosis between the posterior superior alveolar artery and the infraorbital artery. This artery usually has an intraosseous horizontal course along the anterolateral wall of the maxillary sinus at a distance of 18.9 to 19.6 mm from the alveolar ridge.[10] Damage to the alveolar antral artery is a possible complication of maxillary sinus elevation procedures.

Veins and Lymphatic Drainage

Veins arise from the dense venous network of the mucosa and run in different directions accompanying the artery. Part of the venous drainage reaches the cavernous sinus via the infraorbital vein, explaining the potential for extension of maxillary sinus infection to the cavernous sinus.[9]

Lymphatic vessels mainly drain via the ostium into the nasal cavity.[1]

1.2 Endoscopic Anatomy of the Lateral Nasal Wall and Paranasal Sinuses

The lateral nasal wall consists mainly of three constant structures, namely the inferior, middle, and superior turbinates (▶ Fig. 1.6). In some patients a smaller turbinate called the supreme turbinate is also present. The nasal turbinates represent the superomedial delimitation of the respective meati (inferior, middle, superior, and, if present, supreme).

The middle turbinate is the most important to the endoscopic surgeon, representing a crucial landmark for almost all procedures aimed at the ethmoid. The middle turbinate is attached anteriorly to the ethmoidal crest of the maxillary bone. From here, it progresses superomedially to reach the lateral aspect of the lamina cribrosa and then courses posteriorly along the skull base and

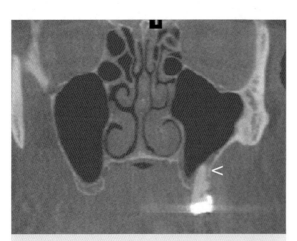

Fig. 1.5 Coronal CT scan showing a thin alveolar bone with a molar root abutting into the maxillary sinus (*arrowhead*), with initial thickening of the sinusal mucosa.

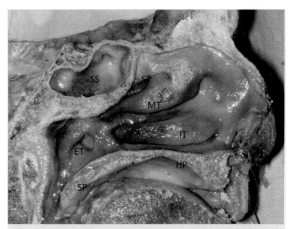

Fig. 1.6 View of the lateral nasal wall. ET, eustachian tube; HP, hard palate; IT, inferior turbinate; MT, middle turbinate; SP, soft palate; SS, sphenoid sinus; ST, superior turbinate; T, tongue.

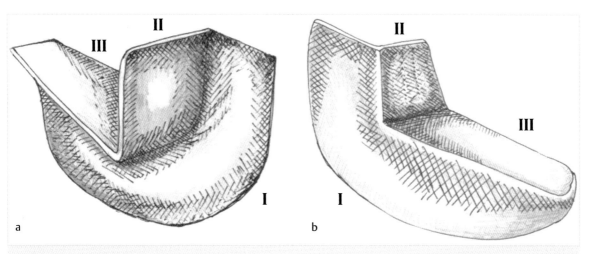

Fig. 1.7 Drawings of the middle turbinate, from (a) an anterior and (b) a posterior point of view. In both drawings the three portions of the middle turbinate, sagittal (I), coronal (II), and axial (III), can be observed. (By kind concession of Dr. M. Bertazzoli.)

inferiorly on the lamina papyracea in an almost coronal plane (vertical portion). Finally, it attaches to the ethmoidal crest of the perpendicular process of the palatine bone.[2] The middle turbinate can therefore be divided into three portions: the first portion, oriented in a sagittal plane, corresponding to the anterior attachment to the skull base; the second, oriented in a coronal plane, attached to the lamina papyracea; and the third, oriented in an axial plane, corresponding to the posterior attachment to the lamina papyracea and palatine bone (▶ Fig. 1.7). The shape of the middle turbinate is highly variable. It can be abnormally pneumatized, in a condition called concha bullosa, or paradoxically curved (▶ Fig. 1.8).

The endoscopic anatomy of the paranasal sinuses is extremely complex. Indeed, the ethmoid sinus consists of air cells adjacent to the superior portion of the lateral nasal wall and the medial wall of the orbit that are often referred to as the *ethmoidal labyrinth*. The number of these cells may vary significantly, from as few as 3 to 18 on each side.[1]

The complexity of these structures is simplified by division of the ethmoidal complex into five parts by four obliquely oriented parallel lamellae, which are easily identifiable during sinus surgery (▶ Fig. 1.9). The first lamella is the uncinate process, the second lamella corresponds to the anterior face of the ethmoidal bulla, the third is the basal (or ground) lamella (attachment of the middle turbinate), and the fourth is the lamella of the superior turbinate. The basal lamella is the most important, since it divides the anterior from the posterior ethmoid. The frontal and maxillary sinuses and the anterior ethmoidal cells drain into the middle meatus, in the area of the ostiomeatal complex, described in Section 1.2.2 (p. 7). The posterior ethmoid cells drain into the superior and supreme meati and then into the sphenoethmoidal recess. The sphenoid sinus drains directly into the sphenoethmoidal recess.

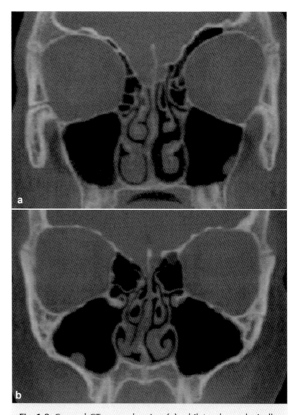

Fig. 1.8 Coronal CT scans showing (a) a bilateral paradoxically curved middle turbinate and (b) a concha bullosa.

1.2.1 Anterior Ethmoid Sinus

The first important structure of the anterior ethmoid is the agger nasi. It can also be seen on anterior rhinoscopy and is located close to the lateral wall, just anteriorly to the middle turbinate insertion. This prominence is very

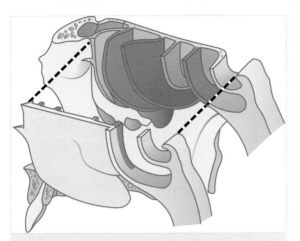

Fig. 1.9 Schematic representation of the four ethmoidal lamellae: (1) uncinate process (*light blue area*); (2) anterior wall of the ethmoidal bulla (*green area*); (3) basal lamella (*purple area*); (4) lamella of the superior turbinate (*blue area*). The anterior wall of the sphenoid sinus (*red area*) and the lamina papyracea (*yellow area*) are also visible.

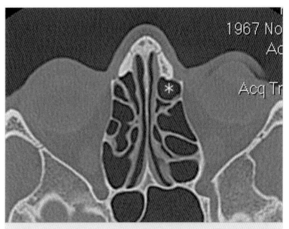

Fig. 1.10 Coronal CT scan showing a left agger nasi cell (*white asterisk*).

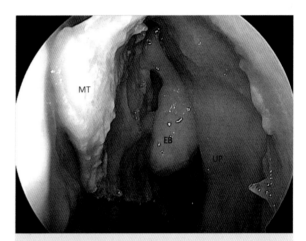

Fig. 1.11 Endoscopic view in a cadaver specimen showing the relationship between the uncinate process (UP), ethmoidal bulla (EB), and middle turbinate (MT).

constant and often pneumatized (70–90% in the literature[3]) by an anterior ethmoidal cell, the agger nasi cell (► Fig. 1.10). The frontal process of the maxilla constitutes the border of this cell anteriorly, the lacrimal bone represents its inferolateral delimitation, the nasal bones its superolateral, and the uncinate process its inferomedial delimitation. The posterior wall of the agger nasi cell constitutes the anterior limit of the frontal recess.

The uncinate process is a thin, sickle-shaped structure, which is part of the ethmoid bone and runs almost in the sagittal plane from anterosuperior to posteroinferior.[11] It is approximately 3 to 4 mm wide and 1.5 to 2 cm in length.[2] Its posterior margin lies parallel to the anterior and inferior surface of the ethmoidal bulla and, together with the bulla, it delimits the semilunar hiatus (► Fig. 1.11). Anteriorly and superiorly, the uncinate process attaches to the ethmoidal crest of the maxilla, just inferior to the attachment of the middle turbinate, and it may be fused with the medial wall of the agger nasi cell. Inferiorly, it is attached to the ethmoidal crest of the inferior turbinate bone and, posteriorly, it is attached to the lamina perpendicularis of the palatine bone.[2] Anteriorly and posteriorly to its attachment to the inferior turbinate bone, the uncinate process has no bony joint, creating the area of the anterior and posterior fontanelles, where the lateral nasal wall consists only of middle meatal mucosa, a layer of connective tissue, and maxillary sinus mucosa. Superiorly and posteriorly, the conformation of the uncinate process may be variable: most commonly (up to 52%) it is attached to the lamina papyracea, but it can also be attached to the skull base or to the middle turbinate (► Fig. 1.12). Sometimes it can divide to connect with different structures simultaneously.[11] The uncinate process forms the anteromedial boundary of the ethmoidal

infundibulum. When it is attached to the lamina papyracea, the superior part of the infundibulum is called the recessus terminalis.

The ethmoidal bulla is the most constant and largest of the anterior ethmoidal cells (► Fig. 1.13). It occupies the middle meatus immediately posterior to the uncinate process and anterior to the basal lamella of the middle turbinate. The bulla is based laterally on the lamina papyracea and has an ostium that opens posteriorly, in front of the basal lamella. In 8% of the subjects, the bulla is not pneumatized, resulting in a bony projection from the lamina papyracea called the torus lateralis. Above and/or behind the bulla, there can be variable air-filled spaces called suprabullar and retrobullar recesses, respectively.[11] These spaces are therefore bordered superiorly by the ethmoidal roof, posteriorly by the basal lamella,

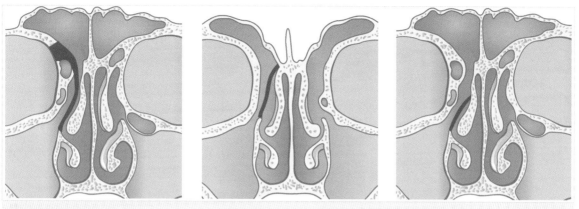

Fig. 1.12 Drawing reproducing the anatomical variations in the superior attachment of the uncinate process.

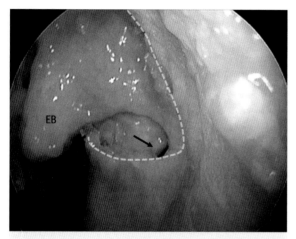

Fig. 1.13 Endoscopic view in the same specimen as shown in ▶ Fig. 1.11. After removal of the uncinate process (section line highlighted by the *yellow line*) a better view of the ethmoidal bulla (EB) is obtained and the natural ostium of the maxillary sinus is exposed (*black arrow*).

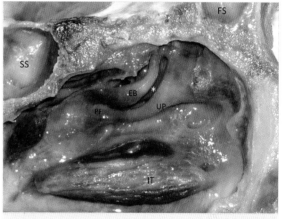

Fig. 1.14 Lateral nasal wall. The semilunar hiatus (*black asterisk*) is located between the ethmoidal bulla (EB) and the uncinate process (UP). Posteriorly to the EB the retrobullar recess is visible (*black arrowhead*). FS, frontal sinus; IT, inferior turbinate; PF, posterior fontanelle; SS, sphenoid sinus.

anteriorly and inferiorly by the posterior wall of the bulla, and laterally by the lamina papyracea, and can communicate superiorly with the frontal recess and semilunar hiatus.[11]

The ethmoidal bulla and uncinate process delimit a two-dimensional cleft called the semilunar hiatus, through which the middle meatus communicates with the ethmoidal infundibulum, a three-dimensional space through which secretions from the anterior ethmoid, the maxillary sinus, and, in some cases, the frontal sinus reach the middle meatus (▶ Fig. 1.14). The superior aspect of the ethmoidal infundibulum is closely related to the frontal recess. When the uncinate process bends laterally to insert onto the lamina papyracea, the upper termination of the ethmoidal infundibulum is called the recessus terminalis. In such cases the frontal sinus drains directly into the middle meatus, medially to the uncinate process. If the uncinate process inserts onto the

skull base or the middle turbinate, the ethmoidal infundibulum is continuous with the frontal recess and therefore the frontal sinus drains into the ethmoidal infundibulum, laterally to the uncinate process. These anatomical variations are responsible for the different patterns of involvement of the paranasal sinuses during rhinosinusitis. Posteroinferiorly, the ethmoidal infundibulum terminates as it empties into the middle meatus and merges with the posterior fontanelle mucosa.[2]

1.2.2 Frontal Sinus

The frontal sinus can vary greatly in shape and degree of pneumatization. Its drainage pathway is extremely complex owing to the possible anatomical variations of the frontal recess. The frontal recess and frontal sinus communicate through the frontal ostium, and, in a sagittal

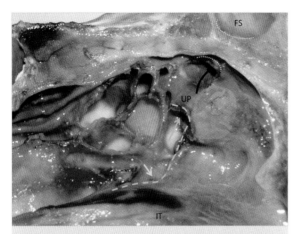

Fig. 1.15 The structure of the frontal recess is determined by the position of the ethmoidal bulla (*blue area*), the agger nasi (*yellow area*), and the uncinate process (UP). In this specimen the frontal ostium (*black arrow*) is located medially to the UP, forming a recessus terminalis (*green arrow*). The hourglasslike appearance of the frontal recess area is highlighted by the *yellow dotted lines*. The *yellow arrow* identifies the maxillary sinus ostium. FS, frontal sinus; IT, inferior turbinate.

Table 1.1 Kuhn's classification of frontal recess and frontal sinus cells

Agger nasi cell	
Supraorbital ethmoid cells	
Frontal cells	
• Type 1	Single frontal recess cell above agger nasi cell
• Type 2	Tier of cells in frontal recess above agger nasi cell
• Type 3	Single massive cell pneumatizing cephalad into frontal sinus
• Type 4	Isolated cell in frontal sinus
Frontal bulla cells	
Suprabullar cells	
Interfrontal sinus septal cell	

Source: Table contents are from Kuhn.[12]

Table 1.2 Modified classification of frontal recess and frontal sinus cells

Agger nasi cell	Cell that is either anterior to the origin of the middle turbinate or sits directly above the most anterior insertion of the middle turbinate into the lateral nasal wall
Frontal ethmoidal cells	Anterior ethmoidal cells that need to be in close proximity to (touching) the frontal process of the maxilla
• Type 1	Single frontal ethmoidal cell above agger nasi cell
• Type 2	Tier of frontal ethmoidal cells above agger nasi cell
• Type 3	Frontal ethmoidal cell that pneumatizes cephalad into the frontal sinus through the frontal ostium but not extending beyond 50% of the vertical height of that frontal sinus on the CT scan that is evaluated
• Type 4	A frontal ethmoidal cell that extends more than 50% of the vertical height of the frontal sinus in the CT scan that is evaluated
Frontal bulla cells	Cells that originate in the suprabullar region but pneumatize into the frontal sinus along its posterior wall
Suprabullar cells	Cells above the ethmoidal bulla that do not enter the frontal sinus
Intersinus septal cell	This cell is associated with the frontal sinus septum and compromises the frontal ostium by occupying part of the opening; it is always medially based and opens into the frontal recess

Source: Data are from Wormald.[13]

plane, they have an hourglasslike appearance, with the narrowest point being the ostium.[2] The main structures that determine the shape and width of the frontal recess are therefore the agger nasi cell, the ethmoidal bulla, and the uncinate process (▶ Fig. 1.15), but different anatomical variations occur when the anterior ethmoid is pneumatized toward the frontal sinus, forming the frontoethmoidal cells. They can be classified as anterior, posterior, lateral, or medial with respect to the frontal ostium, but several classifications have been proposed in the past, the most well known being Kuhn's (▶ Table 1.1).[12] This classification has been significantly modified by Wormald (▶ Table 1.2).[13]

It is now possible to define the concept of an ostiomeatal unit (or ostiomeatal complex), a functional region of the middle meatus located around the uncinate process that includes the uncinate process, ethmoidal infundibulum, anterior ethmoid cells with their ostia, and the ostia of the maxillary and frontal sinuses. An obstruction at this level can be the trigger for disease, potentially involving the whole anterior compartment (frontal sinus, maxillary sinus, anterior ethmoid).

1.2.3 Posterior Ethmoid

The posterior ethmoid is a group of one to five cells located posteriorly to the basal lamella of the middle turbinate that drain into the superior and supreme meati

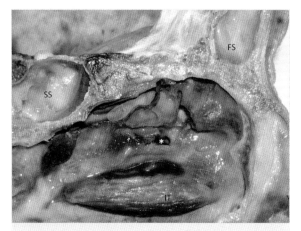

Fig. 1.16 The posterior ethmoid sinus (*yellow area*) is separated from the anterior ethmoid (*blue area*) by the basal lamella (*red dotted line*). The maxillary sinus ostium is visible (*white asterisk*). FS, frontal sinus; IT, inferior turbinate; SS, sphenoid sinus.

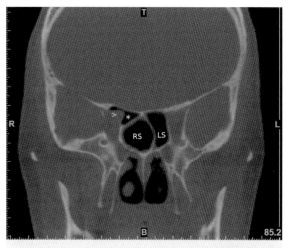

Fig. 1.17 CT scan showing a right Onodi cell (*asterisk*) that contains the optic nerve (*arrowhead*). LS, left sphenoid sinus; RS, right sphenoid sinus.

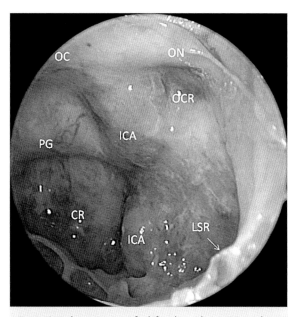

Fig. 1.18 Endoscopic view of a left sphenoid sinus in a cadaver head. CR, clival recess; ICA, internal carotid artery; LSR, lateral sphenoid recess; OC, optic chiasm; OCR, opticocarotid recess; ON, optic nerve; PG, pituitary gland.

(▶ Fig. 1.16). The boundaries of the posterior ethmoid are the basal lamella anteriorly, the anterior sphenoid facet posteriorly (except in the presence of an Onodi cell, described later in this paragraph), the lamina papyracea laterally, and the vertical portion of the superior and supreme turbinates medially. The posterior ethmoid has important relationships with the skull base and the optic nerve, especially in presence of an Onodi cell, a highly pneumatized posterior ethmoidal cell that is lateral and/ or cranial to the sphenoid sinus and usually contains the optic nerve (▶ Fig. 1.17).

1.2.4 Sphenoid Sinus

The sphenoid sinus is located centrally within the skull, in the body of the sphenoid bone. It is bordered laterally by the cavernous portion of the carotid artery and, more superiorly, by the optic nerve. These two structures are separated by the opticocarotid recess. Posteriorly, behind the two sphenoid sinuses, lies the sella turcica containing the pituitary gland (▶ Fig. 1.18). The pneumatization of the sphenoid sinus can be variable and three main types have been described: conchal, presellar, and sellar (▶ Fig. 1.19). The sphenoid sinus drains into the sphenoethmoidal recess, and its natural ostium is located beneath the vertical portion of the superior turbinate, about 10 mm above the choana.

1.2.5 Anterior Skull Base

The lateral aspect of the anterior skull base is composed of the ethmoidal roof, which lies over the ethmoid sinus. Medially, the skull base is composed of the cribriform plate (▶ Fig. 1.20). The ethmoidal roof is superiorly located with respect to the cribriform plate, and a thin bone called the lamina lateralis connects the two structures. The lamina lateralis is the thinnest bone of the skull base and is therefore the site with the highest risk of inadvertent injury during sinus surgery. The cribriform plate and lamina lateralis form an intracranial fossa, called the olfactory fossa, which contains the olfactory bulb and tract. The olfactory fossa has a variable depth, classified by Keros into three groups (▶ Table 1.3).[14]

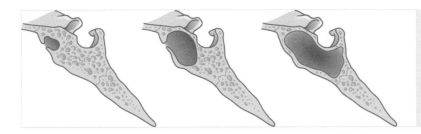

Fig. 1.19 Drawing demonstrating the three main configurations of the sphenoid sinus according to the degree of pneumatization: conchal, presellar, and sellar type.

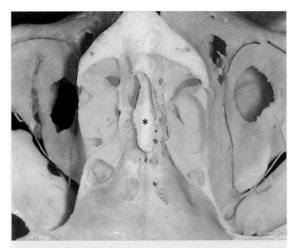

Fig. 1.20 Image of a dry skull showing the relationship between the ethmoidal roof (*yellow area*) and cribriform plate (*green area*). The crista galli (pneumatized in this case, *black asterisk*) separates the two cribriform plates.

Table 1.3 Keros classification of olfactory fossa depth

Type 1	Depth of 1–3 mm
Type 2	Depth of 4–7 mm
Type 3	Depth of 8–16 mm

Source: Data from Keros.[14]

1.3 Microscopic Anatomy of the Sinonasal Mucosa

The sinusal mucosa consists of a pseudostratified ciliated columnar epithelium comprising mainly three types of cells: ciliated cells, goblet cells, and basal cells. Its thickness can vary among the sinuses, from 0.2 to 0.8 mm.[2] The term *pseudostratified* means that, although all the cells are in contact with the basal membrane, the nuclei are not aligned on the same plane, giving the impression of an epithelium composed of several cellular layers. The ciliated cells are columnar epithelial cells with specialized ciliary modifications. At body temperature in the absence of infections, the cilia, located at the apical portions of the cells, beat synchronously 10 to 20 times per second,[15] driving the mucus from the periphery of the sinuses to the natural ostium.[16] When this secretion reaches the nasal cavity and drainage has taken place, it is swallowed and transported into the stomach, where most of pathogenic microbes trapped in the mucus are destroyed.[17] This mechanism is called mucosal clearance. Goblet cells are simple glandular cells whose function is to produce mucus. This production is under the control of the parasympathetic and sympathetic nervous system and is increased after the inspiration of irritating substances or pathogens.[17] Goblet cells in the sinusal cavities are significantly reduced in density compared with the nasal cavities; however, it has been demonstrated that they are more numerous in the maxillary sinus than in the other sinuses.[18] The quantity of mucus produced in the sinuses is adequate to prevent excessive dryness of the epithelium and to create sufficient mucosal clearance.

The basal membrane is located below the epithelium, and beneath the latter there is a thin lamina propria. Basal cells are stem cells located on the basal membrane that do not reach the superficial part of the epithelium. They are able to differentiate into other epithelial cells. Epithelium, basal membrane, and lamina propria constitute the sinusal mucosa, with the lamina propria lying over the submucosal layer (chorion).

The chorion is composed of two layers: the superficial layer consists of dense connective tissue diffusely infiltrated by lymphocytes, while the deeper layer is organized as loose connective tissue, in which the submucosal seromucous glands and the arteries and veins are located. The connective tissue layer adheres to the subjacent periosteum (▶ Fig. 1.21).

In the olfactory region (overlying the cribriform plate, medial surface of the superior nasal concha, and the corresponding opposite septum), a different kind of microscopic anatomy is found. This area is covered by a mucous membrane that is less vascularized than the rest of the nasal mucosa and presents a nonciliated epithelium. It contains the nerve cell bodies that give rise to the olfactory nerve fibers[1] (▶ Fig. 1.22).

1.4 Elements of Physiology

The complexity of the physiological functions of the paranasal sinuses in humans still remains only partially understood. It is assumed that the sinuses play an

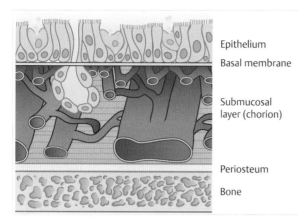

Epithelium

Basal membrane

Submucosal
layer (chorion)

Periosteum

Bone

Fig. 1.21 Schematic representation of the nasal mucosa, consisting of a pseudostratified ciliated epithelium.

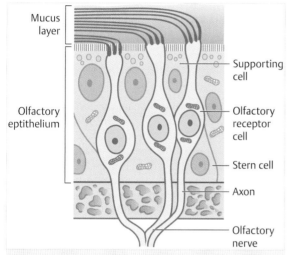

Mucus
layer

Olfactory
eptithelium

Supporting
cell

Olfactory
receptor
cell

Stern cell

Axon

Olfactory
nerve

Fig. 1.22 Schematic representation of the olfactory mucosa.

important role in olfactory and defensive functions, are important for both respiration and phonation, and may participate in reducing skull weight. The mucosa of the paranasal sinuses is continuous with the nasal mucosa and represents one of the first defensive barriers of the respiratory tract. As described in Section 1.3 (p.10), its epithelium is covered by a layer of mucus produced by goblet cells and glands of the submucosal layer. This secretion is considered the first line of defense.[19]

1.4.1 Mucus

The mucus is composed of two different layers. The inferior thin layer (called sol) is produced by the microvilli of the pseudostratified columnar cells and envelops the cilia, allowing them to move. The upper layer is a gel produced by goblet cells and submucosal glands, and one of its main functions is to offer an insertion point for the tips of the cilia.[17] The mucus entraps bacteria and inhaled particles and, by the process of mucociliary clearance, is driven toward the nasal cavity and finally into the stomach.[20]

1.4.2 Defensive Role of the Sinonasal Mucosa

The sinus mucosa is an active element that responds to external and pathological stimuli with many different and specialized reactions. For example, the secretion of mucus increases during upper respiratory tract infections. This mucus, through the synchronous beating of the cilia at approximately 12 Hz,[15] is transported following well-defined pathways from the sinusal cavities to the nose and pharynx. Nitric oxide (NO) is known to be the main regulator of ciliary beat and its production may increase during inflammation or infections.[21] As described in Section 1.4.1 (p.11), mucociliary clearance allows mucus, in which inhaled particles or bacteria are trapped, to be drained through the ostium; this mechanism generally preserves sinusal sterility.[22,23]

Other factors including pH, oxygen supply, humidity, temperature, ionic balance, O_2 and CO_2 concentrations also contribute to regulation of the ciliary beat rate, therefore influencing the efficiency of mucociliary clearance. Pollution (i.e., smoke, dust, and several chemical elements) may also influence mucociliary clearance directly, by damaging the mucosa, or indirectly, by modifying the chemical and physical characteristics of the mucus. This reduction in the efficiency of mucociliary clearance increases the susceptibility to infection or neoplastic diseases of the upper airway.[24]

In addition, the nasal mucosa has immunological functions, both *adaptive* and *innate*. Adaptive immunity, mediated by B and T lymphocytes, is characterized by its specificity and memory. Conversely, innate immunity is mediated by macrophages and leukocytes, which are commonly known to nonspecifically engulf pathogens; however, innate immunity also has considerable specificity and the ability to discriminate between pathogens and self.[25] Mechanisms of action of innate immunity are

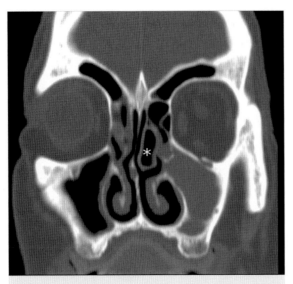

Fig. 1.23 CT scan showing a left concha bullosa (*asterisk*) with left maxillary sinus dysventilation.

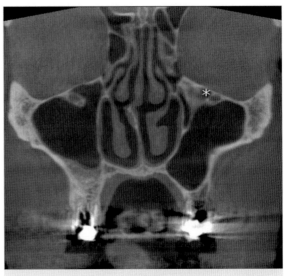

Fig. 1.24 CT scan showing a left Haller cell (*asterisk*) closing the maxillary sinus drainage pathway with mild mucosal thickening.

based on the production of different molecules; some of these are involved in chemoattraction and activation of the innate and adaptive system cells, while others inhibit microbial proliferation and direct microbicidal activity. The most important molecules are lysozyme, lactoferrin, defensin and cathelicidin, and secretory leukocyte proteinase inhibitor.

1.5 Pathophysiological Implications of Nasal and Sinusal Ventilation

The nose acts as an air conditioner, warmer, filter, and humidifier. The spontaneous congestion and decongestion of the nasal venous sinuses causes an asymmetric airflow between the two nasal fossae,[26] alternating over a period of 2 to 4 hours.[27,28] This phenomenon is called the *nasal cycle*, and it divides the workload of air conditioning so that while one nasal cavity works, and is exposed to potential pathogens, the other has a resting period during which it can recover.

The airflow patterns during normal quiet respiration highlight a main flow stream in the middle airway and middle meatus. No significant differences have been reported between inspiration and expiration, but in the latter phase the maximum velocity is lower.[29]

Physiologically, exhaled and inhaled air does not come into direct contact with the sinusal mucosa. Indeed, there is no significant direct airflow from the nasal cavities into the sinusal cavities, especially during inhalation. With regard to the maxillary sinus, its natural ventilation is remarkably slow, following a diffusion-dominated pattern. This limited ventilation may be protective for the sinus, preventing mucosal drying, maintaining sterility with high NO concentrations, and minimizing entry of pathogens.[30] However, the presence of an accessory ostium causes alterations in local flow patterns inside the maxillary sinus, producing a transit stream through the flow path connecting the natural and accessory ostia.[31] This small bypass flow, enhancing sinus ventilation, reduces the NO concentration in the sinus. Therefore, whereas ventilation is necessary, excessive ventilation due to an accessory ostium or very large ostium (i.e., after middle meatal antrostomy) may not be clinically beneficial, because it could increase the washout of NO, which has bacteriostatic and mucociliary regulatory properties, increase the access of pathogens into the sinus, and cause mucosal drying.[30] However, proper patency of the natural ostium of the maxillary sinus and other paranasal sinuses is of utmost importance in maintaining a healthy sinusal mucosa.

Anatomical conditions that can promote dysventilation of the ostiomeatal complex and consequently of the maxillary sinus are the marked pneumatization of an agger nasi cell, frontoethmoidal cells, and/or the ethmoidal bulla, the presence of concha bullosa[32] (▶ Fig. 1.23) or a Haller cell (▶ Fig. 1.24), and variation in the shape and dimensions of the uncinate process (i.e., lateralization or pneumatization). These conditions may increase the rate of postoperative complications after maxillary sinus grafting procedures. Functional endoscopic sinus surgery (FESS) is the mainstay of treatment for such conditions and can also be performed in conjunction with oral surgery. Please see Chapter 7 (p. 128) for further details.[33] Septal deformities can also reduce ventilation of the middle meatus and ostiomeatal complex and predispose to sinusal diseases; indeed, septal surgery is reported to be indicated in patients needing endoscopic sinus surgery for chronic sinusitis, whether or not this is of dental origin.[34]

1.6 Pathophysiology of Odontogenic Rhinosinusitis

Odontogenic maxillary sinusitis may be triggered by perforation or irritation of Schneider's membrane, as the physiologically sterile maxillary sinus may become contaminated by oral pathogens when a perforation occurs. See Chapter 4 (p.66) for details of microbial contamination. This condition may be a consequence of dental pathoses such as severe periodontitis, pulpitis, caries, or complications of a dental procedure, whether traditional or related to an implant or maxillary sinus elevation.[35] See Chapter 3 (p.40) for details of clinical scenarios.

Spontaneous resolution of an acute odontogenic sinusitis is frequently seen in a normally ventilated maxillary sinus. In the case of maxillary dysventilation, the defense mechanisms of the sinusal mucosa may be insufficient to restore normal conditions within the sinus and the inflammatory and infectious processes may become chronic and involve the ethmoid, the frontal, and in some cases, the sphenoid sinuses.[36]

Key Points

- The maxillary sinus is a large air-filled cavity within the body of the maxilla, lined with mucoperiosteum (also called *Schneider's membrane*).
- The anatomical relationship between the maxillary sinus and the teeth is highly variable, depending on maxillary pneumatization of the alveolar process.
- The lateral nasal wall consists of three nasal turbinates, namely the inferior, middle, and superior turbinates, which delimit superomedially the inferior, middle, and superior meati. The middle turbinate is the most important to the endoscopic surgeon, representing a crucial landmark for almost all ethmoidal procedures.
- The sinusal mucosa is a pseudostratified ciliated columnar epithelium composed of three main types of cells: ciliated cells, goblet cells, and basal cells.
- The mucociliary clearance mechanism transports mucus from the periphery of the sinuses, through the natural ostium to the nasal cavity, and then to the stomach, where particles and bacteria entrapped in the mucus are destroyed.

References

[1] Janfaza P, Montgomery WW, Salman SD. Nasal cavities and paranasal sinuses. In: Janfaza P, Nadol JB, Galla RJ, Fabian RL, Montgomery WW, eds. Surgical Anatomy of the Head and Neck. Philadelphia, PA: Lippincott Williams and Wilkins; 2001:259–318

[2] Kennedy DW, Bolger WE, Zinreich SJ. Diseases of the Sinuses: Diagnosis and Management. Hamilton, Ontario: BC Decker; 2001

[3] Lund VJ, Stammberger H, Fokkens WJ et al. European position paper on the anatomical terminology of the internal nose and paranasal sinuses. Rhinol Suppl 2014; 24: 1–34

[4] Wormald PJ, ed. Endoscopic Sinus Surgery: Anatomy, Three-Dimensional Reconstruction, and Surgical Technique. New York, NY: Thieme; 2004

[5] Wang L, Gun R, Youssef A et al. Anatomical study of critical features on the posterior wall of the maxillary sinus: clinical implications. Laryngoscope 2014; 124: 2451–2455

[6] Underwood AS. An inquiry into the anatomy and pathology of the maxillary sinus. J Anat Physiol 1910; 44: 354–369

[7] Robinson S, Wormald PJ. Patterns of innervation of the anterior maxilla: a cadaver study with relevance to canine fossa puncture of the maxillary sinus. Laryngoscope 2005; 115: 1785–1788

[8] Becker AM, Hwang PH. Surgical anatomy and embryology of the maxillary sinus and surrounding structures. In: Duncavage JA, Becker SS, eds. The Maxillary Sinus: Medical and Surgical Management. New York, NY: Thieme; 2011:1–7

[9] Lang J, ed. Clinical Anatomy of the Nose, Nasal Cavity and Paranasal Sinuses. Stuttgart: Georg Thieme Verlag; 1989

[10] Maridati P, Stoffella E, Speroni S, Cicciu M, Maiorana C. Alveolar antral artery isolation during sinus lift procedure with the double window technique. Open Dent J 2014; 8: 95–103

[11] Stammberger HR, Kennedy DW Anatomic Terminology Group. Paranasal sinuses: anatomic terminology and nomenclature. Ann Otol Rhinol Laryngol Suppl 1995; 167: 7–16

[12] Kuhn FA. Chronic frontal sinusitis: the endoscopic frontal recess approach. Operative Techniques in Otolaryngol Head and Neck Surg 1996; 7: 222–229

[13] Wormald PJ, ed. Endoscopic Sinus Surgery: Anatomy, Three-Dimensional Reconstruction, and Surgical Technique. 3rd ed. New York, NY: Thieme; 2013

[14] Keros P. On the practical value of differences in the level of the lamina cribrosa of the ethmoid [in German] Z Laryngol Rhinol Otol 1962; 41: 809–813

[15] Wanner A. Clinical aspects of mucociliary transport. Am Rev Respir Dis 1977; 116: 73–125

[16] Proctor DF. The mucociliary system. In: Proctor DF, Anderson I, eds. The Nose: Upper Airway Physiology and the Atmospheric Environment. Amsterdam: Elsevier; 1982: 352–376

[17] Bailey BJ, Calhoun KH, Derkay CS, et al, eds. Head and Neck Surgery: Otolaryngology. Philadelphia, PA: Lippincott Williams and Wilkins; 2001

[18] Tos M. Goblet cells and glands in the nose and paranasal sinuses. In: Proctor DF, Anderson I, eds. The Nose: Upper Airway Physiology and the Atmospheric Environment. Amsterdam: Elsevier; 1982:155–162

[19] Drettner B. The paranasal sinuses. In: Proctor DF, Anderson I, eds. The Nose: Upper Airway Physiology and the Atmospheric Environment. Amsterdam: Elsevier; 1982: 145–162

[20] Waguespack R. Mucociliary clearance patterns following endoscopic sinus surgery. Laryngoscope 1995; 105 Suppl 71: 1–40

[21] Lundberg JO, Farkas-Szallasi T, Weitzberg E et al. High nitric oxide production in human paranasal sinuses. Nat Med 1995; 1: 370–373

[22] Rohr AS, Spector SL. Paranasal sinus anatomy and pathophysiology. Clin Rev Allergy 1984; 2: 387–395

[23] Abou-Hamad W, Matar N, Elias M et al. Bacterial flora in normal adult maxillary sinuses. Am J Rhinol Allergy 2009; 23: 261–263

[24] Levine HL, Pais Clemente M, eds. Sinus Surgery: Endoscopic and Microscopic Approaches. New York, NY: Thieme; 2005

[25] Ramanathan M Jr, Lane AP. Innate immunity of the sinonasal cavity and its role in chronic rhinosinusitis. Otolaryngol Head Neck Surg 2007; 136: 348–356

[26] Eccles R. Nasal airflow in health and disease. Acta Otolaryngol 2000; 120: 580–595

[27] Stoksted P. Rhinometric measurements for determination of the nasal cycle. Acta Otolaryngol Suppl 1953; 109: 159–175

[28] Flanagan P, Eccles R. Spontaneous changes of unilateral nasal airflow in man: a re-examination of the 'nasal cycle'. Acta Otolaryngol 1997; 117: 590–595

[29] Chung SK, Kim SK. Digital particle image velocimetry studies of nasal airflow. Respir Physiol Neurobiol 2008; 163: 111–120

[30] Rennie CE, Hood CM, Blenke EJSM et al. Physical and computational modeling of ventilation of the maxillary sinus. Otolaryngol Head Neck Surg 2011; 145: 165–170

[31] Na Y, Kim K, Kim SK, Chung SK. The quantitative effect of an accessory ostium on ventilation of the maxillary sinus. Respir Physiol Neurobiol 2012; 181: 62–73

[32] Zinreich SJ, Mattox DE, Kennedy DW, Chisholm HL, Diffley DM, Rosenbaum AE. Concha bullosa: CT evaluation. J Comput Assist Tomogr 1988; 12: 778–784

[33] Felisati G, Borloni R, Chiapasco M, Lozza P, Casentini P, Pipolo C. Maxillary sinus elevation in conjunction with transnasal endoscopic treatment of rhino-sinusal pathoses: preliminary results on 10 consecutively treated patients. Acta Otorhinolaryngol Ital 2010; 30: 289–293

[34] Poje G, Zinreich JS, Skitarelić N et al. Nasal septal deformities in chronic rhinosinusitis patients: clinical and radiological aspects. Acta Otorhinolaryngol Ital 2014; 34: 117–122

[35] Lechien JR, Filleul O, Costa de Araujo P, Hsieh JW, Chantrain G, Saussez S. Chronic maxillary rhinosinusitis of dental origin: a systematic review of 674 patient cases. Int J Otolaryngol 2014; 2014: 465173

[36] Saibene AM, Pipolo GC, Lozza P et al. Redefining boundaries in odontogenic sinusitis: a retrospective review evaluation of extramaxillary involvement in 315 patients. Int Forum Allergy Rhinol 2014; 4: 1020–1023

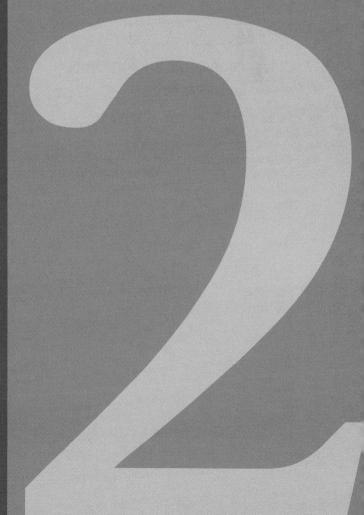

Chapter 2

Imaging of the Maxilla and Paranasal Sinuses

2 Imaging of the Maxilla and Paranasal Sinuses

Roberto Maroldi and Andrea Borghesi

Contents Overview

The purpose of this chapter is to describe the role of radiological imaging in the assessment and prevention of sinonasal complications following dental treatment. The chapter is divided into three sections. The first section introduces general aspects of imaging techniques such as panoramic radiography, periapical radiography, and CT. The second section presents a series of high-quality images illustrating radiological anatomy of the maxilla and paranasal sinuses. The third section focuses on the specific role of radiological imaging in the clinical decision-making process.

2.1 Techniques of Radiological Examination

The radiological techniques used in the study of maxillofacial region disorders are intraoral radiography, panoramic radiography, lateral cephalometric projection, CT, and MRI. These diagnostic tools differ significantly in their technical characteristics, acquisition modalities, and indications. Panoramic radiography, periapical radiography, and CT are the most commonly used techniques in the evaluation and prevention of sinonasal complications after dental treatment.

2.1.1 Panoramic Radiography

Principles and Technique

Panoramic radiography is a diagnostic tool that captures, in a single two-dimensional image, the curved layer of teeth, jaws, surrounding structures, and tissue. The basic principles of panoramic radiography are similar to those of conventional tomography.[1] In order to obtain, in one single image, a radiographic projection of the maxillary and mandibular dental arches, which

have a curved morphology, a dedicated panoramic X-ray machine is needed. This radiographic machine consists of two main parts: the X-ray tube and image receptor that rotate around the head of the patient at the same time but at different speeds (the image receptor is slower than the X-ray tube).[1,2] This acquisition modality ensures that only one curved layer of the jaws is in focus (the so-called image layer).[1–3] In panoramic radiography, only the structures lying within the image layer (thickness 1–3 cm) are captured with good definition, while the other structures are geometrically distorted, blurred, enlarged, or diminished.[1–3] Accurate patient positioning is, therefore, critical in order to obtain a diagnostic image (i.e., both teeth and jaws within the image layer). Correct positioning requires that the patient should be standing up straight with the head immobilized in a forehead and/or chin rest, the Frankfurt plane should be parallel to the floor, the midsagittal plane centered, and the incisors resting on a notch of radiolucent bite block.[1,2] All foreign objects in the maxillofacial region, including dentures, piercings, glasses, earrings, necklaces, etc., should be removed before starting the acquisition process.[1,2] Moreover, the patient should place his tongue in close contact with the hard palate and hold it there during the exposure in order to avoid, on the final image, a radiolucent area above the maxillary alveolar process (▶ Fig. 2.1).

In addition, considering the relatively long data acquisition time (15–20 seconds), the cooperation of the patient is very important, and he or she should remain absolutely still for the entire acquisition process.

In accordance with previously reported data[1] we do not use a lead apron in our clinical routine, especially in children and patients with short neck, because it may interfere with machine movement and produce artifacts during the exposure, significantly compromising the image quality.

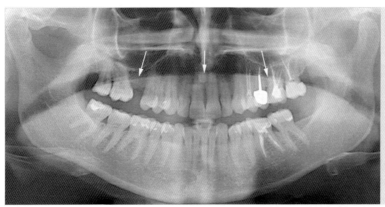

Fig. 2.1 Panoramic radiograph showing a radiolucent band projected above the maxillary alveolar process because the tongue (*arrows*) was not placed against the palate during the exposure.

Errors and Artifacts

Panoramic radiography is considered to be a relatively simple radiological technique, although the image quality obtained with this method is not always sufficiently accurate to evaluate the teeth, maxilla, and mandible, especially in the hands of an inexperienced operator.[4] In fact, Rushton et al[5] observed that the poor quality of panoramic radiographs is mostly due to a lack of knowledge of the basic requirements for producing a diagnostic image, especially in relation to correct patient positioning. The most frequent positioning error is incorrect positioning of the patient's tongue. This error, which occurs in up to 46% of cases,[4] produces a radiolucent band (the palatoglossal space) projected onto the maxillary alveolar process (▶ Fig. 2.1).

The second most frequent error, in up to 26% of cases, is the superimposition of the cervical spine. This produces a large radiopaque band projected over the anterior jaws, because the neck of the patient is angled forward.

Other common but less frequently observed patient positioning errors[1,2] are:
- Head too far forward: incisors appear blurred and narrowed.
- Head too far back: incisors appear blurred and magnified.
- Head tilted downward: the occlusal plane is too curved (looks like it is smiling) and the anterior mandibular roots are outside the image layer (shorter and blurred).
- Head tilted upward: the occlusal plane is flattened (with a "frowning" configuration), the anterior maxillary roots are outside the image layer (blurred), and their apices may overlap with the hard palate.
- Head rotated: the posterior structures on the side toward which the head is rotated are magnified in the horizontal dimension.

Indications, Advantages, and Disadvantages of Panoramic Radiography

Panoramic radiography is widely used in daily routine as a first-choice diagnostic tool for dental and maxillofacial evaluation. It provides information on lesions within the jaws in addition to the relationships of anatomical structures such as the alveolar crest, the maxillary sinus, and the nasal floor.[6]

The main indications for panoramic radiography are:
- Periapical and periodontal disease.
- Presence or absence of residual tooth roots.
- Third molar position.
- Trauma or fractures.
- Cysts and tumors.
- Preliminary preimplant evaluation of the height of residual alveolar bone.[7]
- Postoperative evaluation of implant treatment.

The advantages of panoramic radiography are:
- Large anatomical area covered.
- Relatively low radiation dose (10 times less than a full-mouth intraoral survey).[8]
- Relatively fast and easy to perform.
- Suitable for patients unable to open their mouths.

The disadvantages of panoramic radiography are:
- Image quality decreases in noncooperative patients.
- Lower spatial resolution than intraoral radiography.
- Structures outside image layer appear blurred and distorted.
- Vertical and horizontal magnifications (more pronounced in posterior areas) that vary between different panoramic units.[6,8–10]
- Objects with high density produce typical ghost artifacts on the opposite side of the film (magnified and blurred) that may hide or obscure important anatomical structures (▶ Fig. 2.2).

2.1.2 Intraoral Periapical Radiography

Intraoral radiography, routinely used in general dental practice, still remains the prevalent imaging modality for evaluating the teeth and surrounding structures. Intraoral radiographs can be divided into three categories: periapical, bitewing, and occlusal radiographs. These

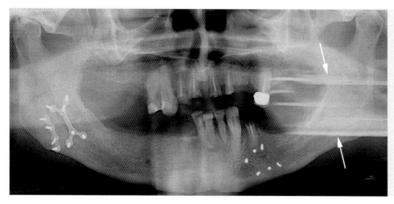

Fig. 2.2 Surgical plates and screws located on the right mandibular ramus produce ghost artifacts on the left side of the image (*arrows*).

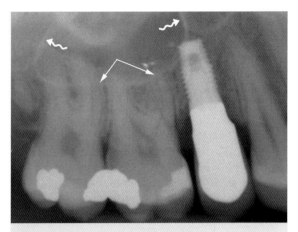

Fig. 2.3 Intraoral periapical radiograph of the maxillary premolar and molar regions, showing the maxillary sinus floor (*arrows*) and septa within the maxillary sinus (*wavy arrows*).

radiographic images are obtained by placing the image receptor intraorally. Periapical radiography captures an image of a limited region of the jaws and, as the name suggests, it should include the crown and roots of the teeth and the surrounding periapical bone (▶ Fig. 2.3).

The main indications of this technique include:

- Detection of dental caries.
- Detection of periapical and periodontal disease.
- Evaluation of root morphology before extraction, endodontic treatment, and postoperative assessment of implants.

A bitewing image includes only the crowns of the teeth and the adjacent alveolar crest and is mainly used to detect interproximal caries and to assess the initial stages of periodontal disease. An occlusal image is a planar radiograph used to provide a view of a large section of the jaws and is sometimes used to determine the buccolingual extension of pathological conditions.

Two intraoral projection techniques may be used for periapical radiography: the paralleling technique and the bisecting angle technique.[11,12] The paralleling technique is the method of choice because it produces images with less distortion and reduces the radiation exposure of the patient.[11,12] In the paralleling technique, also called the long-cone technique, the image receptor has to be placed in the mouth of the patient, parallel to the long axis of the tooth, and the central beam of the X-ray tube head needs to be directed at right angles to both the tooth and the receptor. However, considering the morphology of the dental arches and the alveolar process, the image receptor cannot be placed in direct contact with the tooth. To reduce the magnification caused by this separation, the X-ray source should be located relatively far from the teeth. This distant positioning minimizes geometric distortion and allows the teeth and surrounding structures to be represented on the image very close to

the actual size. The main advantage of the paralleling technique is that it provides accurate and reproducible images with minimal geometric distortion and little magnification. The main disadvantage of this technique is the position of the image receptor, which may be very uncomfortable for some patients.

The bisecting angle technique is applied when anatomical configuration or lack of patient cooperation precludes the paralleling technique. In the bisecting angle technique the image receptor is placed as close to the tooth as possible, and the central beam of the X-ray is directed perpendicular to an imaginary line bisecting the angle formed between the long axis of the tooth and the long axis of the image receptor. The main advantage of the bisecting angle technique is the position of the image receptor, which is more comfortable for patients in all regions of the mouth. The main disadvantage of this technique is the distortion of the image due to the angulation of the X-ray beam.

In some instances (e.g., pediatric patients and those with a disability) conventional intraoral radiography is not suitable.[12] For these patients, who are unable to tolerate the intraoral placement of the image receptor, an alternative technique is extraoral periapical radiography.[13-15] This technique is more comfortable for patients and provides images with adequate diagnostic quality[13-15]; however, it cannot be considered as a substitute for conventional intraoral radiography owing to its lower spatial resolution and because it cannot be used to examine the anterior teeth.[13]

2.1.3 Cone Beam and Multidetector Computed Tomography

Computed tomography (CT) is an X-ray diagnostic imaging technique that generates high spatial resolution images of a particular anatomical volume, differentiating the various organs and tissues according to the different absorption rates of the X-ray beam that passes through the patient. The amount of X-ray energy absorbed depends on the density of the tissue, and the X-ray beam exiting the patient is captured and electronically converted by detectors into digital images. These images consist of small volumetric units (called voxels) and the computer assigns to each voxel a grayscale value (ranging from white to black) representing tissue density. Therefore, on the final digital image, cortical bone is white, water is mid-gray, and air is black.

There are two main CT techniques commonly used in the evaluation of maxillofacial disease (including sinonasal disease) in daily clinical routine: multidetector CT (MDCT) and cone beam CT (CBCT). Both CT modalities produce images with isotropic voxels (i.e., voxels of equal length in all three dimensions); this means that images have similar spatial resolution in all planes, allowing high-quality multiplanar (MPR) and three-dimensional reconstructions. However, these CT methods differ in technology, mode and time of acquisition, radiation dose, spatial and contrast resolution, and intensity of metal artifacts.[16–18]

Technology

MDCT scanners consist of an X-ray tube that emits a collimated, fan-shaped X-ray beam directed to a variable number of linear detector rows mounted on a rotating gantry. Conversely, CBCT units consist of an X-ray tube that emits a pyramidal or cone-shaped X-ray beam directed toward a two-dimensional flat panel detector.

Acquisition

The acquisition time of a CBCT examination is highly variable and depends on the type of scanner used, the field of view (FOV), and the exposure parameters selected. Typically, the time required to scan the entire maxillofacial region, using full FOV CBCT units, ranges from 20 to 40 seconds. Conversely, the time needed to acquire the same anatomical region using last generation MDCT scanners is significantly shorter and no longer than 8 seconds.

This time difference between CBCT and MDCT acquisition is very important, especially when examining very young children and elderly patients, who can be noncooperative. In these situations in particular, the long acquisition time of CBCT scanners may increase the risk of motion artifacts, reducing image quality.

The position of the patient during the CT scan represents another difference between the two methods. In MDCT scanners, the patient lies supine on the CT table. In CBCT units, depending on the type of machine used, patients may be scanned in three possible positions: sitting, standing, or supine. It should be noted that vertical positioning of the patient (standing or sitting) requires secure immobilization of the head in order to prevent motion artifacts.[18]

Radiation Dose

One of the major advantages of CBCT in comparison with MDCT is the reduction in radiation dose. The effective radiation dose of CBCT units varies depending on the type and model of CBCT scanner, FOV selected, and exposure time.[19,20] It is important to emphasize that the effective radiation dose can be reduced because CBCT devices employ a pulsatile X-ray beam. In fact, in CBCT the actual exposure time corresponds to a fraction of the acquisition time.[20]

Many published reports have analyzed the effective dose delivered by different CBCT units. These studies include one of the most important in maxillofacial imaging, which showed that the effective dose of CBCT devices (range 13–82 µSv) was significantly lower than that of MDCT devices (range 474–1160 µSv).[21]

Based on the dosimetric implications of these data, and when clinically indicated, CBCT may be considered the diagnostic tool of choice, particularly in young and cooperative patients. However, it should be noted that the marked difference in effective dose between CBCT and MDCT may be significantly reduced using appropriate low-dose protocols.[22,23]

Spatial Resolution

Another advantage that makes CBCT a particularly attractive technique is its higher spatial resolution compared with MDCT. This specific feature represents a valuable addition to the assessment of the maxillofacial region. In a recently published study, Pauwels et al[24] demonstrated that CBCT scans outperform MDCT for visualization of small, high-contrast structures. In fact, this advantage of CBCT over MDCT is seen mainly in the study of the fine anatomical details of the maxilla, mandible, and paranasal sinuses (such as fossae, foramina, canals, and recesses) (▶ Fig. 2.4).

Contrast Resolution

One of the main disadvantages of CBCT compared with MDCT scans is the low contrast resolution, which is not suitable for soft tissue contrast discrimination. It has been reported in the literature that, for head and neck imaging, the CBCT unit has a soft tissue contrast discrimination approximately 10 times lower than that of MDCT.[16]

In addition, the Hounsfield scale, generally used to measure tissue density in CT, is not calibrated on CBCT because the different grayscale value assigned to each voxel depends on its density and position in the image volume. This makes CBCT units unreliable for comparing tissue density based on CT number. Moreover, CBCT is not suitable for evaluating the extension of pathological disorders into soft tissues and precludes the possibility of using intravenous contrast media.[18] Therefore, in order to assess the extension of a lesion in the soft tissues, MDCT or, even better, MRI are the tools of choice. In fact, MRI is the diagnostic method with the highest contrast resolution, making it the most suitable technique for soft tissue evaluation.

Metal Artifacts

Artifacts caused by metal objects, such as metallic restorations, crowns, root canal filling materials, brackets, implants, surgical plates, and screws, remain a challenge in CT imaging.

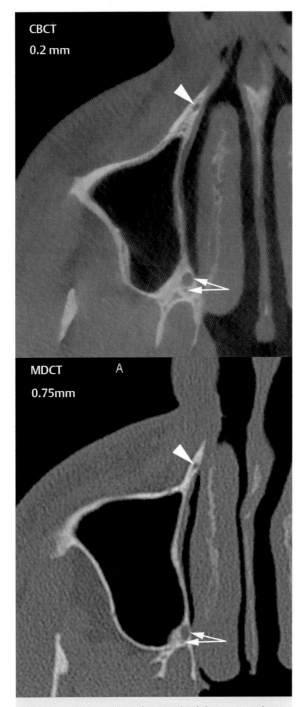

Fig. 2.4 Axial CT images at the same level demonstrate that cone-beam computed tomography (CBCT; top) is superior to multidetector computed tomography (MDCT; bottom) in the detection of fine anatomical details. The anterior superior alveolar canal (*arrowhead*) and palatine canals (*arrows*) are shown.

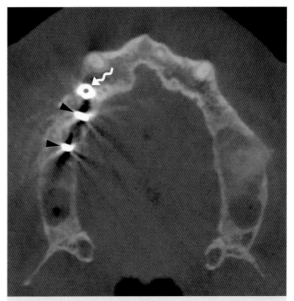

Fig. 2.5 Axial CBCT image at the level of the maxillary alveolar process shows metal artifacts caused by a dental implant (*wavy arrow*) and screws (*arrowheads*).

Reports in the literature suggest that these artifacts are less prominent in CBCT than in MDCT.[23,25]

However, the effects of metal artifacts on CBCT image quality (i.e., beam hardening, scattering, quantum noise, and photon starvation) are similar to those observed in MDCT. In both CT techniques metal artifacts may mask or, more frequently, alter the representation of structures located near metallic objects (▶ Fig. 2.5), reducing the diagnostic value of the images. For this reason, the structures located close to a metal object should be carefully analyzed in order to avoid interpretation errors.[26]

Several published reports have analyzed different methods for metal artifact reduction (including adapted scanning protocols, specific reconstruction algorithms, or postprocessing techniques). However, the possibilities of further reduction on CBCT images without increasing exposure parameters (such as increasing the mAs, kVp, exposure time, and FOV size) are actually limited.[26]

Postprocessing

In the evaluation of the maxilla and paranasal sinuses, the high-resolution volumetric data set produced by CT scans (CBCT or MDCT) is postprocessed, generating multiple reconstruction images (MPR) in different planes (such as axial, coronal, and sagittal), usually ≤ 1 mm in

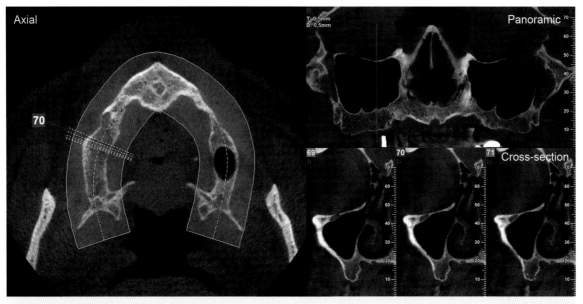

Fig. 2.6 Multiplanar reconstruction images of maxilla obtained with Dentascan software.

thickness. In addition, using dedicated reconstruction software for dental arches (Dentascan), the data set is further processed in MPR reconstructions (usually 0.5 or 1 mm thick) that are either parallel (Panorex) or perpendicular (cross) to the curvature of the maxillary alveolar process (▶ Fig. 2.6). These reconstructions allow a more detailed evaluation of the maxillary alveolar process and its relationships with the maxillary sinus and the floor of the nasal cavity.

2.2 Radiological Anatomy of the Maxilla and Paranasal Sinuses

An adequate knowledge of the imaging anatomy of the maxilla, nasal cavity, and maxillary sinus is of the utmost importance, particularly when dealing with the evaluation and prevention of sinonasal complications of dental treatment. Radiological examination of the maxilla, nasal cavity, and paranasal sinuses may be accomplished with a wide variety of techniques (i.e., periapical radiography, panoramic radiography, MDCT, and CBCT). These diagnostic tools, in particular CBCT, provide detailed information of this anatomical area.

In this section, a series of high-quality radiographic and CBCT images is presented, illustrating the anatomy of the maxilla, nasal cavity, maxillary sinus, and ostiomeatal complex (▶ Fig. 2.7, ▶ Fig. 2.8, ▶ Fig. 2.9, ▶ Fig. 2.10, ▶ Fig. 2.11, ▶ Fig. 2.12, ▶ Fig. 2.13, ▶ Fig. 2.14, ▶ Fig. 2.15, ▶ Fig. 2.16, and ▶ Fig. 2.17).

2.3 Role of Imaging in the Evaluation and Prevention of Sinonasal Complications following Dental Treatment

2.3.1 Introduction

Odontogenic sinusitis is a well-known condition and the literature reports that 10 to 12% of cases of maxillary sinusitis are attributed to an odontogenic source.[27] However, odontogenic sinusitis is probably underestimated. In fact, more recent publications suggest that up to 30 to 40% of maxillary sinus infections have a dental origin.[28]

The maxillary sinus is the largest sinonasal cavity, and is located between the nasal and oral cavities. Its floor separates the sinus from the tooth roots and is made of dense cortical bone. The floor is formed by the alveolar process, which is highly variable in thickness, particularly when comparing dentulous and edentulous subjects.[27] Furthermore, the apical aspects of the tooth roots may protrude into the sinus without a bony covering (i.e., covered only by Schneider's membrane),[27,28] particularly when the maxillary sinus is significantly pneumatized. The close anatomical relationship of the maxillary sinus to the dentoalveolar unit promotes the development of odontogenic infections into the sinus. Infections occur when Schneider's membrane is irritated or perforated by conditions such as periapical abscesses, periodontal disease, dental trauma, or iatrogenic causes such as tooth extraction, endodontic treatment, implant placement,

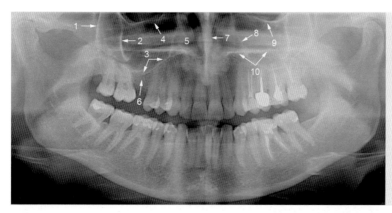

Fig. 2.7 Panoramic radiograph. 1, lateral maxillary sinus wall; 2, zygomatic process; 3, maxillary sinus floor; 4, infraorbital canal; 5, inferior turbinate; 6, maxillary alveolar process; 7, nasal septum; 8, medial maxillary sinus wall; 9, orbital floor; 10, hard palate.

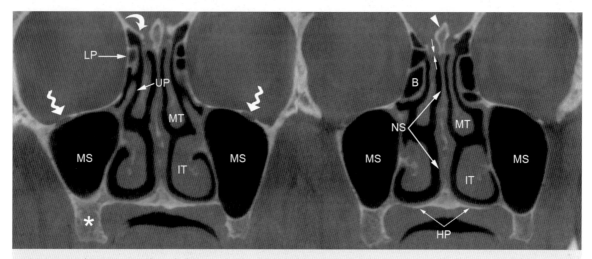

Fig. 2.8 Coronal CBCT images through the anterior ethmoidal labyrinth, showing the infraorbital canal (*wavy arrow*), fovea ethmoidalis (*curved arrow*), maxillary alveolar process (*asterisk*), crista galli (*arrowhead*), and cribriform plate (*opposing arrows*). B, ethmoidal bulla; HP, hard palate; IT, inferior turbinate; LP, lamina papyracea; MS, maxillary sinus; MT, middle turbinate; NS, nasal septum; UP, uncinate process.

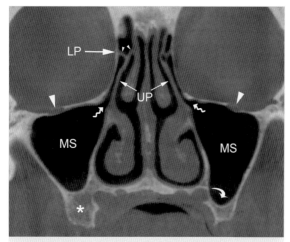

Fig. 2.9 Coronal CBCT image at the level of the insertion of the uncinate process. The infraorbital canal (*arrowhead*), maxillary sinus ostium (*wavy arrow*), maxillary alveolar process (*asterisk*), insertion of the uncinate process (*small arrowheads*), and alveolar recess of the maxillary sinus (*curved arrow*) can be seen. LP, lamina papyracea; MS, maxillary sinus; UP, uncinate process.

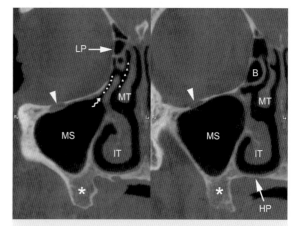

Fig. 2.10 Cross-sectional CBCT images at the level of the ostiomeatal complex, showing the infraorbital canal (*arrowhead*), maxillary sinus ostium (*wavy arrow*), ethmoidal infundibulum (*dotted line*), middle meatus (*small triangles*), and maxillary alveolar process (*asterisk*). B, ethmoidal bulla; HP, hard palate; IT, inferior turbinate; LP, lamina papyracea; MS, maxillary sinus; MT, middle turbinate.

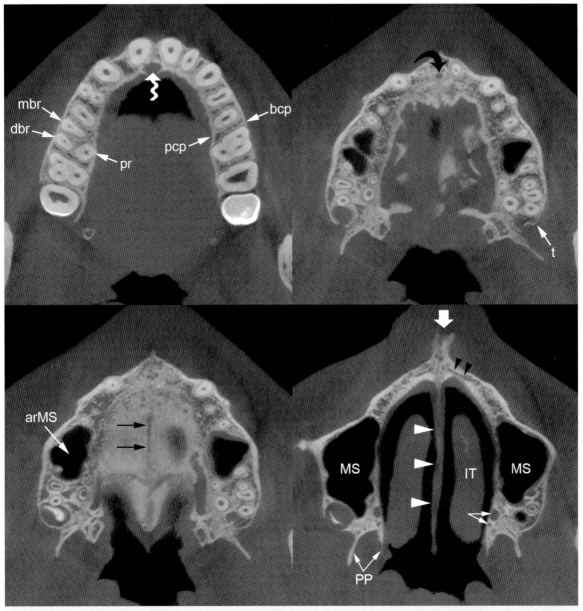

Fig. 2.11 Axial CBCT images at the level of the maxillary alveolar process, showing the incisive foramen (*wavy arrow*), mesial buccal root (mbr), distal buccal root (dbr), palatal root (pr), palatal cortical plate (pcp), buccal cortical plate (bcp), incisive canal (*curved arrow*), maxillary tuberosity (t), alveolar recess of maxillary sinus (arMS), intermaxillary suture (*black arrows*), anterior nasal spine (*large arrow*), anterior superior alveolar canal (*small black arrowheads*), nasal septum (*large arrowheads*), and palatine canals (*small arrows*). IT, inferior turbinate; MS, maxillary sinus; PP, pterygoid plates.

and maxillary sinus augmentation.[29] Odontogenic sinusitis is usually considered to be limited to the maxillary sinus; however, a recently published study found that this was the case in only 40.3% of patients with odontogenic sinusitis.[30]

The accurate diagnosis of sinusitis originating from an odontogenic source is important because the pathophysiology, microbiology, and treatment differ from sinusitis caused by other conditions.[27] In particular, the management of odontogenic sinusitis often requires treatment of the sinonasal infection as well as the dental cause of infection.[27] For this reason, radiological imaging is an important tool in making the correct diagnosis, and is helpful in assessing the extent of the sinonasal infection. Imaging can also provide useful anatomical information of dentoantral relationships in the prevention of sinonasal accidents and complications during and following various dental treatments.

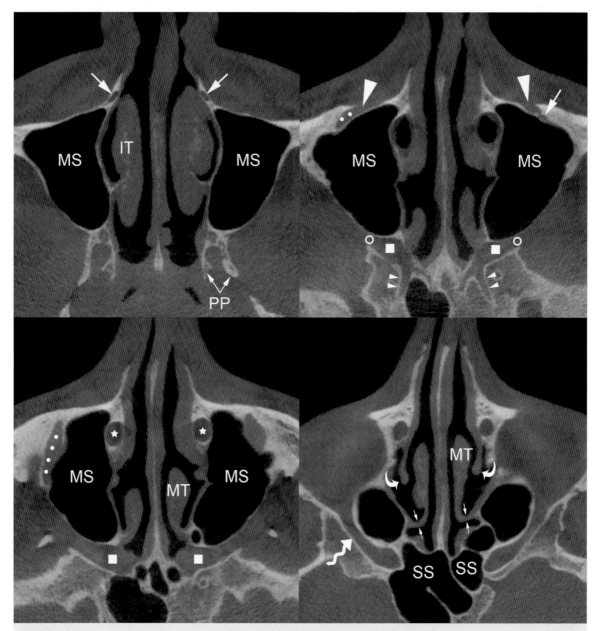

Fig. 2.12 Axial CBCT images at the level of the maxillary sinuses. The anterior superior alveolar canal (*arrow*), infraorbital canal (*dotted line*), infraorbital foramen (*large arrowheads*), pterygopalatine fossa (*square*), pterygomaxillary fissure (*open circle*), vidian canal (*small arrowheads*), nasolacrimal duct (*star*), uncinate process (*small curved arrow*), basal lamella of the middle turbinate (*small opposing arrows*), and inferior orbital fissure (*wavy arrow*) are visible. IT, inferior turbinate; MS, maxillary sinus; MT, middle turbinate; PP, pterygoid plates; SS, sphenoid sinus.

2.3.2 Role of Imaging in the Evaluation of Sinonasal Complications after Dental Treatment

The most common cause of odontogenic sinusitis is iatrogenic and, in a recent systematic review, this accounted for 65.7% of cases.[31] The iatrogenic causes of sinusitis include tooth extraction, root canal treatment, dental implant placement, maxillary sinus augmentation, and maxillary orthognathic surgery.[27–29] The accidental displacement of roots (during extraction), endodontic filling materials (used in root canal obturation), and dental implants into the maxillary sinus is a relatively common complication in dental clinical practice and can cause sinusitis by triggering an inflammatory response and interrupting mucociliary clearance.[31,32] Therefore, when a

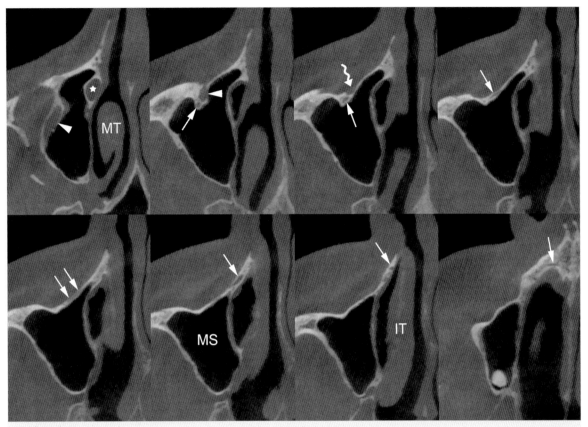

Fig. 2.13 Axial CBCT images show the course of the anterior superior alveolar canal (*arrows*) along the anterior maxillary sinus wall. Also visible are the infraorbital canal (*arrowheads*), infraorbital foramen (*wavy arrow*), and nasolacrimal duct (*star*). IT, inferior turbinate; MS, maxillary sinus; MT, middle turbinate.

patient presents with sinusitis after dental treatment, imaging is essential in differentiating between sinusitis caused by obstructed drainage pathways and odontogenic disease. Failure to identify the dental origin of infection may lead to recurrent sinusitis.[33]

The radiological techniques available in patients with suspected odontogenic sinusitis include periapical radiography, panoramic radiography, and CT (MDCT and CBCT).

Periapical radiography is the standard diagnostic tool to assess periapical periodontitis and it is considered an essential part of the diagnosis and treatment of endodontic disease.[34] In addition, if peri-implantitis is suspected, periapical projections may be used to detect bone loss resulting in peri-implant radiolucencies. In an in vitro study, Mengel et al[35] found that CBCT was superior to periapical radiography in the detection of peri-implant defects and more accurate in the delineation of their three-dimensional extent. However, in this study the simulated peri-implant bone defects were large (4 mm thick).

Conversely, Dave et al[36] showed recently that digital long-cone periapical radiography has excellent sensitivity (100%) and specificity (98.9%) in the detection of small

peri-implant bone defects (no more than 0.675 mm thick) and that its accuracy was better than CBCT (sensitivity ranged from 64.4 to 97.8% and specificity ranged from 67.8 to 97.8%). The authors of this study suggest that the superior performance of digital long-cone periapical radiography is probably due to its better resolution, contrast, and detail of bone quality than CBCT.[36] Moreover, the accuracy and precision of CBCT can be reduced by the presence of metal artifacts, which may make small bone defects more difficult to detect.[36] However, it should be remembered that periapical radiographs have the limitation of a two-dimensional view: focal bone defects located on buccal or palatal surfaces may be missed.

A second limitation of periapical radiographs is again related to the two-dimensional view: periapical radiolucencies and maxillary sinus involvement is frequently underestimated, especially in the posterior maxilla.[37]

Panoramic radiography produces a flat representation of the curved surfaces of the jaws and is a more useful diagnostic tool than periapical radiography for providing an overview of the maxillary sinus and evaluating the anatomical relationships between the alveolar bone and teeth, the floors of the maxillary sinuses, and the nasal cavities.[38] This technique is usually helpful for detecting

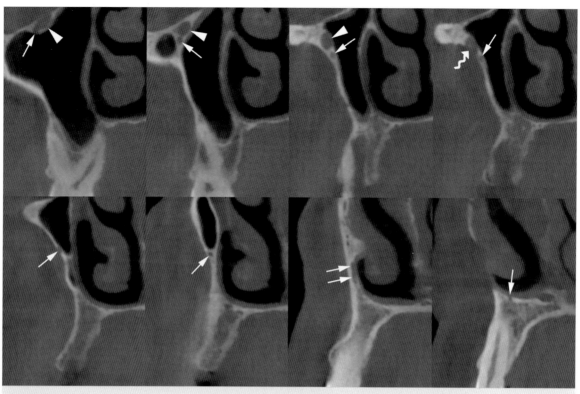

Fig. 2.14 Cross-sectional CBCT images demonstrate that the anterior superior alveolar canal (*arrows*) originates from infraorbital canal (*arrowheads*) and runs toward the midline through the anterior wall of the maxillary sinus. The infraorbital foramen (*wavy arrow*) is also seen.

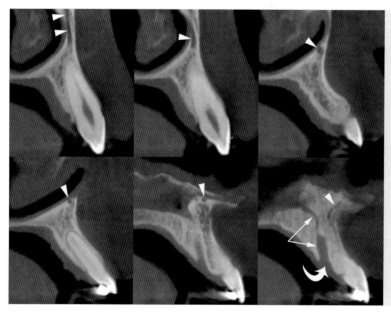

Fig. 2.15 Cross-sectional CBCT images show the vertical course of the nasopalatine canal (*arrows*) and its inferior opening, the incisive foramen (*curved arrow*). In the midline area, the anterior superior alveolar canal (*arrowheads*) may be located in close proximity to the nasopalatine canal.

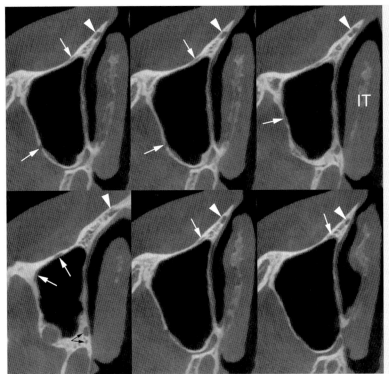

Fig. 2.16 Axial CBCT images demonstrate the course of the posterior superior alveolar canal (*arrows*) along the lateral and anterior maxillary sinus walls. The anterior superior alveolar canal (*arrowheads*), palatine canals (*small black arrows*), and inferior turbinate (IT) are also detected.

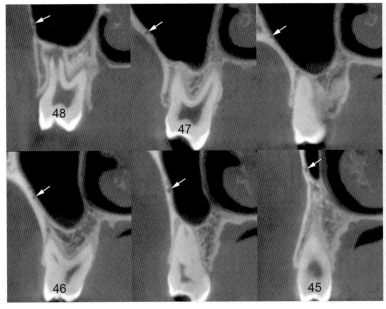

Fig. 2.17 Cross-sectional CBCT images show the intraosseous location of the posterior superior alveolar canal (*arrows*) and its relationship to the alveolar ridge and maxillary sinus in the molar/premolar region. 45, second premolar; 46, first molar; 47, second molar; 48, third molar.

mucosal thickening, mucous retention cysts, sinus opacification, periapical lesions, displaced roots, or foreign bodies within the sinuses[27,38] (▶ Fig. 2.18). However, the overlap of anatomical structures (such as the hard palate), patient positioning errors, the horizontal and vertical magnification, and the two-dimensional nature limit the usefulness of this examination for detailed assessment of the maxillary alveolar bone and sinonasal cavities. In fact, the lack of any cross-sectional information makes panoramic radiography insufficient to estimate the true relationship between the floor of the sinonasal cavities and the tooth roots or dental implants that project into the sinus air space (▶ Fig. 2.19). Furthermore, in oroantral communications, a relatively common complication of

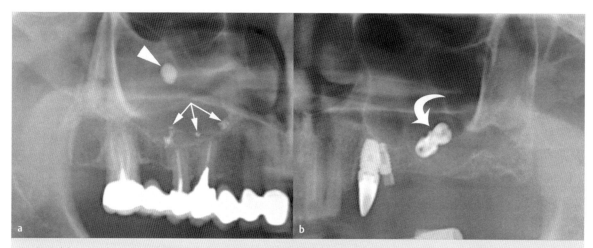

Fig. 2.18 (a) Cropped panoramic radiograph shows opacification of the right maxillary sinus. A well-defined radiopaque mass, referred to as an antrolith (*arrowhead*), is identified within the maxillary sinus. Endodontic filling material (*arrows*) projected along the maxillary sinus floor is also observed. (b) Cropped panoramic radiograph shows an implant dislocated into the inferior part of the maxillary sinus (*curved arrow*).

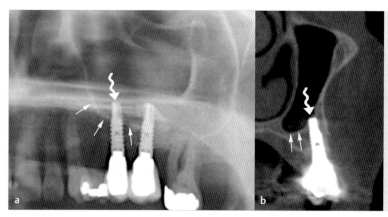

Fig. 2.19 (a) Cropped panoramic radiograph shows a dental implant (*wavy arrow*) projected over the floor of the maxillary sinus (*arrows*). (b) Cross-sectional CBCT image of the same patient demonstrates the true position of the implant (*wavy arrow*) and its relationship with the maxillary sinus floor (*arrows*).

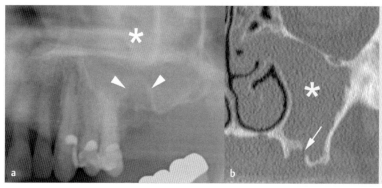

Fig. 2.20 Chronic maxillary sinusitis after tooth extraction. (a) Cropped panoramic radiograph shows opacification of the left maxillary sinus (*asterisk*) and the socket after extraction of the first molar (*arrowheads*). (b) Coronal MDCT image detects a focal interruption of the maxillary sinus floor at the site of tooth extraction (*arrow*); the maxillary sinus is filled with inflammatory material (*asterisk*).

dental treatment (mainly detected after tooth extraction),[39] small bony defects in the sinus floor are rarely diagnosed radiographically (▶ Fig. 2.20).

For these reasons, CT is considered the gold standard for diagnosing odontogenic sinusitis, owing to its ability to visualize sinonasal cavities with high-resolution images. The CT data set obtained during axial acquisition can be postprocessed to produce multiple two-dimensional MPR images. These MPR images allow three-dimensional views of maxillofacial anatomy, without superimposition of structures outside the volume of interest, and can provide precise information about the dental disease within the maxilla and its relationship with surrounding anatomical structures such as sinonasal cavities, canals, fossae, and foramina.

Nowadays, CBCT is becoming the diagnostic tool of choice in the study of the inflammatory changes in the nasal and paranasal sinus mucosa, in particular when a dental cause of sinusitis is suspected. For this indication, CBCT has gradually replaced MDCT because it provides images using a lower radiation dose and with higher spatial resolution (≤200 μm) and fewer metal artifacts than MDCT.[17,18] For these reasons, the image quality of CBCT is considered superior to MDCT for detection of the odontogenic origin of sinusitis and changes in the sinonasal mucosa.[18,40,41] Furthermore, CBCT images provide detailed information on the ostiomeatal complex and frontal sinus drainage anatomy prior to functional endoscopic sinus surgery, even when the inflammatory process involves the ethmoid and frontal sinuses.

However, the main drawback of CBCT is its poor contrast resolution, which precludes soft tissue evaluation and contrast medium injection.[18,41] Therefore, when an orbital (usually secondary to ethmoiditis) or intracranial (usually secondary to frontal sinusitis) complication is suspected, MDCT is the first-choice technique.

Odontogenic sinusitis may be chronic or acute. In both cases, odontogenic origin of infection occurs when Schneider's membrane is damaged by conditions arising from the dentoalveolar unit. Chronic sinusitis is frequently associated with mucosal thickening (more than 4 mm), sinus opacification, reactive bone sclerosis, and thickening of the sinus walls (► Fig. 2.21a). In contrast, fluid collection is the finding that most closely correlates with acute sinusitis (► Fig. 2.21b). Bearing in mind that CT cannot demonstrate sinus membrane perforation, the findings that may indicate an increased risk of developing sinusitis after dental treatment are:

- Endodontic filling material extending into periapical tissue or into the sinus cavity.[42]
- Persistent periapical disease after incomplete endodontic therapy (► Fig. 2.22).
- Oroantral communication[27,39] (► Fig. 2.23).
- Dental implants protruding more than 4 mm into the sinonasal cavities [43,44] (► Fig. 2.24).
- Displaced roots or foreign bodies within the sinonasal cavities[32] (► Fig. 2.25).
- Peri-implant bone defects[31] (► Fig. 2.26, ► Fig. 2.27).
- Bone graft infection (► Fig. 2.28) or graft displacement within the sinus after maxillary sinus augmentation.[45]

Maxillary fungus ball is another complication that may occur after endodontic treatment. It may be observed more frequently when the tooth roots indent the sinus floor. In fact, the literature reports that endodontic

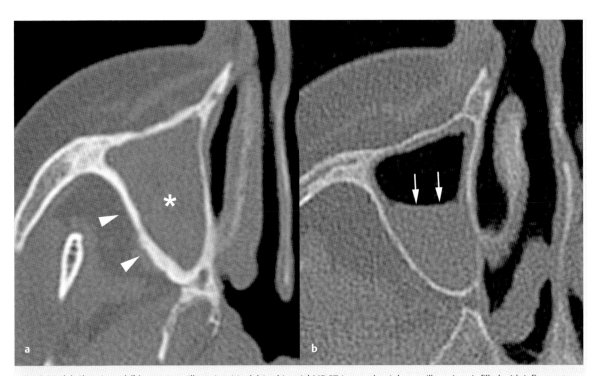

Fig. 2.21 (a) Chronic and (b) acute maxillary sinusitis. (a) In this axial MDCT image the right maxillary sinus is filled with inflammatory material (*asterisk*); reactive sclerosis and thickening of the lateral sinus wall (*arrowheads*), secondary to chronic inflammation, are also observed. (b) Axial MDCT image shows an air–fluid level within the right maxillary sinus (*arrows*), representing acute infection.

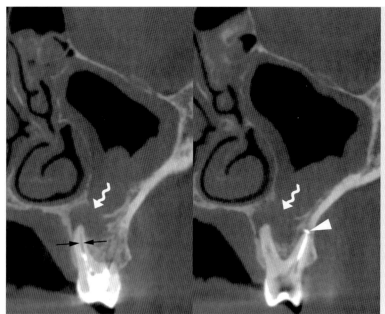

Fig. 2.22 Maxillary sinusitis after improper endodontic therapy. Cross-sectional CBCT images detect a large area of bone resorption around the palatal root of a maxillary molar tooth after incomplete root canal treatment (*opposing arrows*). The floor of the maxillary sinus is interrupted (*wavy arrow*) with significant thickening of the adjacent mucosa. The buccal root canal is overfilled (*arrowhead*).

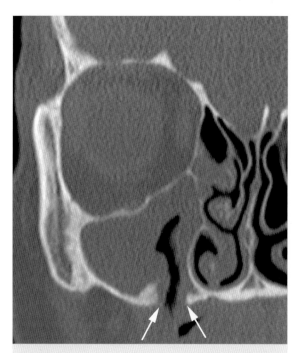

Fig. 2.23 Coronal MDCT image detects an oroantral communication (*arrows*) with maxillary sinusitis following dental implant failure.

The CT findings of maxillary fungus ball depend on the high content of heavy metals (iron and manganese) and calcium within fungal hyphae. As a result, an "ironlike density" and/or scattered microcalcifications within the sinus may be detected (▶ Fig. 2.29). Sinus opacification, bone sclerosis, and thickening of the sinus walls are also observed in maxillary fungus ball (▶ Fig. 2.29). In one study,[48] the prevalence of ironlike density in maxillary fungus ball was 71.9%, whereas the prevalence of microcalcifications was 16.3%.

The location of the ironlike density and calcifications in maxillary fungus ball is almost always central within the sinus (▶ Fig. 2.29). Conversely, foreign bodies (such as endodontic material and dental implants) and calcifications in nonfungal maxillary sinusitis tend to have a different intrasinus location. Maxillary sinus foreign bodies may be located at the periphery (more frequently near the sinus floor) (▶ Fig. 2.18 and ▶ Fig. 2.30b) or near the maxillary ostium (carried by mucociliary clearance) (▶ Fig. 2.25). Calcifications in nonfungal sinusitis are generally located at the periphery,[49] near the sinus walls (often within the thickened submucosal layer) (▶ Fig. 2.30a and ▶ Fig. 2.31).

2.3.3 Role of Imaging in the Prevention of Complications

According to the literature, iatrogenic causes are the most common etiological factors in odontogenic sinusitis.[31] Therefore, in order to avoid unnecessary complications following dental treatment (such as implant placement and maxillary sinus augmentation), a preoperative radiological assessment of the maxilla, nasal cavity, and maxillary sinus anatomy is essential, because of the close

treatment of maxillary teeth is an important risk factor for developing fungus ball.[46,47] Furthermore, a relatively recent publication showed that endodontic therapy is more frequently associated with maxillary fungus ball than chronic sinusitis.[47] These observations reinforce the hypothesis that the zinc oxide contained in root-filling materials promotes fungal proliferation.

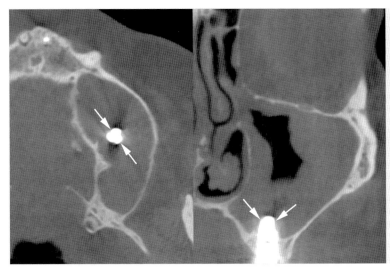

Fig. 2.24 Axial (left) and coronal (right) CBCT images show significant mucosal thickening around the part of the implant protruding into the maxillary sinus cavity (*arrows*).

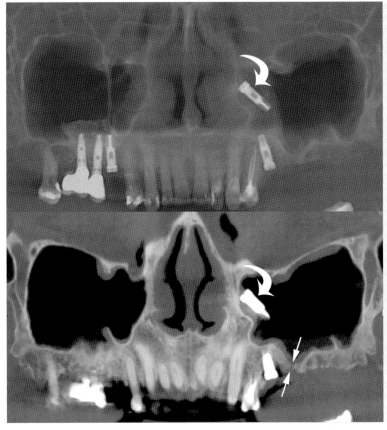

Fig. 2.25 Panoramic CBCT images, with 20 mm (top) and 0.5 mm (bottom) slice thickness, demonstrate migration of a dental implant into the left maxillary sinus (*curved arrows*). A focal interruption of the sinus floor is also detected (*arrows*).

anatomical relationship of the dentoalveolar unit to the floor of the maxillary sinus and the nasal cavity.

Panoramic radiography is the most commonly used radiological technique in preliminary evaluation of crestal alveolar bone and the cortical boundaries of the maxillary sinus and nasal cavity. However, this technique has significant limitations as a definitive preoperative planning tool because of its two-dimensional nature. For

example, it is well known that panoramic projections of the posterior maxilla underestimate the amount of bone available for the implant placement procedure, and therefore they may overestimate the need for sinus augmentation. Moreover, Shiki et al[38] recently showed that the detection rate of anatomical variations and lesions of the maxillary sinus (such as pneumatization, septa, mucosal thickening, and mucous retention cysts) on

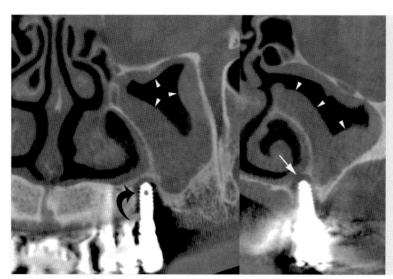

Fig. 2.26 Peri-implantitis and sinusitis. Panoramic (left) and cross-sectional (right) CBCT images detect a peri-implant bone defect (*curved arrow*) with focal interruption of the nasal cavity floor (*arrow*). Circumferential mucosal thickening in the left maxillary sinus is also observed (*arrowheads*).

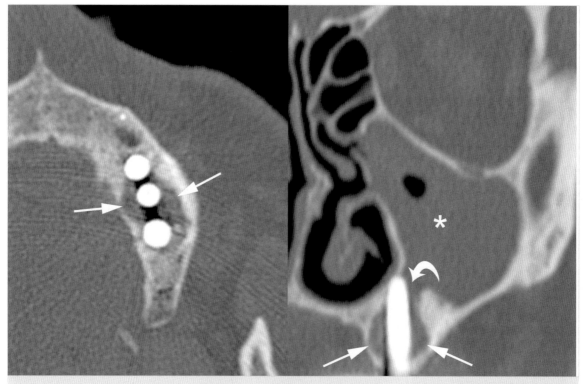

Fig. 2.27 Peri-implantitis and sinusitis after maxillary sinus augmentation. Axial (left) and coronal (right) MDCT images. A large bone defect is seen around the implant (*arrows*); the floor of the left maxillary sinus is interrupted (*curved arrow*) and the sinus is filled with inflammatory material (*asterisk*).

panoramic radiographs was significantly lower than the detection rate on CBCT. The detection of these anatomical variations and lesions within the sinus is very important in predicting the risk of sinonasal complications. In fact, the assessment of maxillary sinus pneumatization is crucial before tooth extraction, endodontic treatment, or implant placement. The presence of septa within the sinus increases the risk of sinus membrane perforation during sinus augmentation procedures.[50] Similarly, the presence of mucosal thickening on preoperative CT imaging increases the risk of late chronic sinusitis after sinus floor augmentation.[45] Conversely, mucous retention cysts (submucosal pseudocystic lesions), one of the most common benign pathologies and frequently detected on CT (▶ Fig. 2.32), are not always a contraindication for sinus grafting.[51]

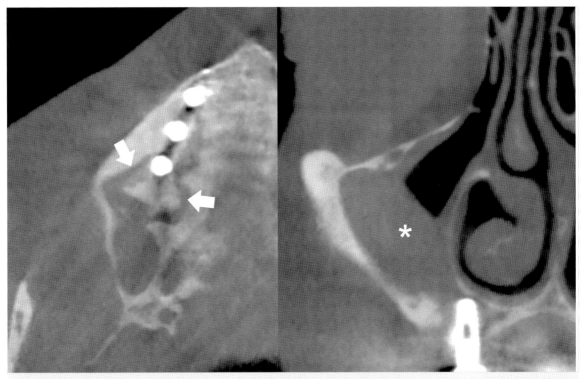

Fig. 2.28 Bone graft infection and sinusitis after maxillary sinus augmentation. Axial (left) and coronal (right) CBCT images demonstrate an osseointegration failure of the graft (*large arrows*) with right maxillary sinusitis (*asterisk*).

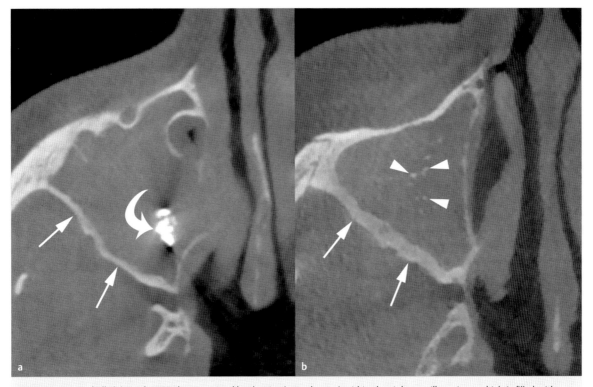

Fig. 2.29 Fungus ball. **(a)** Axial CBCT shows an ironlike density (*curved arrow*) within the right maxillary sinus, which is filled with inflammatory material. Thickening of the sinus walls (*arrows*) suggests chronic inflammation. **(b)** In axial CBCT, the right maxillary sinus is filled by inflammatory material with scattered microcalcifications (*arrowheads*). Reactive changes (thickening and sclerosis) of the sinus walls are clearly depicted (*arrows*).

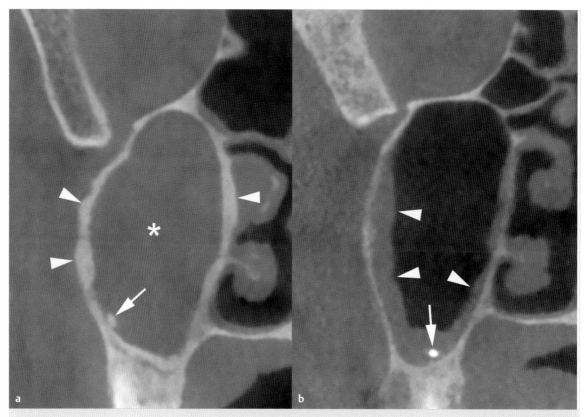

Fig. 2.30 (a) Calcification in nonfungal sinusitis. Cross-sectional CBCT image shows a nodular calcification (*arrow*) located at the periphery of the right maxillary sinus, which is filled with inflammatory material (*asterisk*). Sclerosis and thickening of the sinus walls (*arrowheads*) suggests chronic inflammation. (b) Maxillary foreign body. Cross-sectional CBCT image demonstrates a nodular hyperdense material (endodontic filling material) located near the sinus floor (*arrow*) and mild mucosal thickening (*arrowheads*).

For these reasons, CBCT is now the preferred method for preoperative assessment, in particular before implant placement and sinus augmentation procedures.

During implant placement, dentists usually avoid critical structures such as the maxillary sinus, nasal cavity, and incisive canal.

In sinus grafting, surgeons need to pay attention to the neurovascularization of the maxilla. This detailed information is provided preoperatively by CBCT. In fact, the high spatial resolution of CBCT is able to detect two important neurovascular channels (diameter ≤ 1 mm) occupied by neurovascular units and located in the bony walls of the maxillary sinus: the anterior and posterior superior alveolar canals.[52,53] The anterior superior alveolar canal passes across the maxillary bone in the infraorbital region (▶ Fig. 2.13, ▶ Fig. 2.14, and ▶ Fig. 2.15). The posterior superior alveolar canal passes along the lateral and anterior walls of the maxillary sinus (▶ Fig. 2.16 and ▶ Fig. 2.17). Axial and cross CBCT images accurately detect and follow the course of both channels in the bony walls. Damage to these neurovascular channels during surgical procedures can cause neurovascular complications and may lead to perforation of Schneider's membrane.

Finally, it should be mentioned that CT assessment of ostiomeatal complex patency is mandatory in order to prevent intraoperative and postoperative sinusitis after sinus floor elevation procedures (▶ Fig. 2.10).

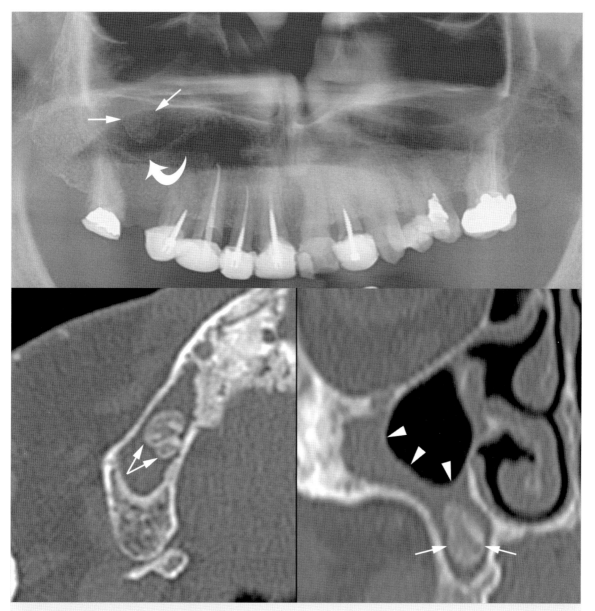

Fig. 2.31 Ossification in nonfungal sinusitis. Panoramic radiograph (top) shows a well-defined radiopaque lesion (*arrows*) projected over the floor of the right maxillary sinus (*curved arrow*). The regular shape, thin cortical rim, and internal mineralized pattern indicate an ossified structure. Axial and coronal MDCT images (bottom) demonstrate two ossified lesions located near the inferior wall of the sinus (*arrows*), within the thickened submucosal layer (*arrowheads*).

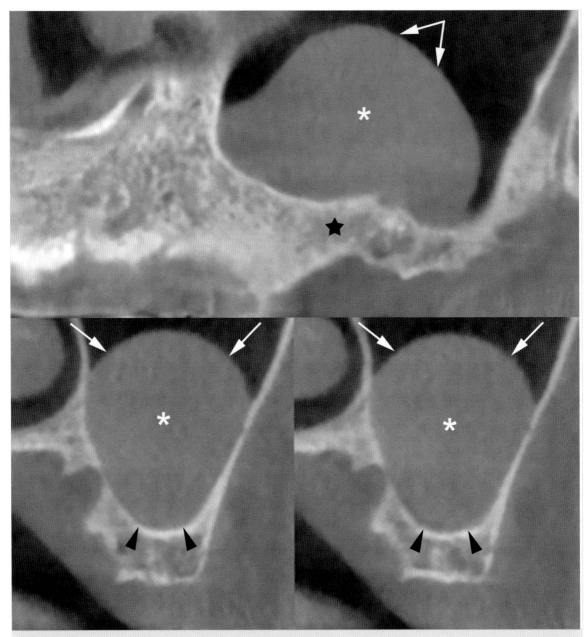

Fig. 2.32 Mucous retention cyst. In cropped panorex (top) and cross (bottom) CBCT images, the left maxillary sinus is partially filled by a hypodense lesion (*asterisk*) attached to the alveolar recess (*arrowheads*). The lesion shows a convex shape and smooth borders (*arrows*). No bone changes are observed, particularly at the site of attachment (*arrowheads*). The maxillary alveolar process (*star*) is also shown.

Key Points

- Panoramic radiography, periapical radiography, and CT are the most commonly used techniques in the evaluation and prevention of sinonasal complications after dental treatment.
- CT is considered the gold standard in the evaluation and management of inflammatory sinonasal disease. For this indication, in particular when a dental origin of sinusitis is suspected, CBCT has gradually replaced MDCT.
- The preoperative detection of anatomical variations and lesions of the maxillary sinus (such as pneumatization, septa, course of the superior alveolar canals, mucosal thickening, and mucous retention cysts) is very important in predicting the risk of sinonasal complications following dental treatment. For this indication, CBCT is the diagnostic tool of choice.
- The CT assessment of ostiomeatal complex patency is mandatory before maxillary sinus augmentation.

References

[1] Murray D, Whyte A. Dental panoramic tomography: what the general radiologist needs to know. Clin Radiol 2002; 57: 1–7

[2] Boeddinghaus R, Whyte A. Dental panoramic tomography: an approach for the general radiologist. Australas Radiol 2006; 50: 526–533

[3] Riecke B, Friedrich RE, Schulze D et al. Impact of malpositioning on panoramic radiography in implant dentistry. Clin Oral Investig 2015;19:781–790.

[4] Akarslan ZZ, Erten H, Güngör K, Celik I. Common errors on panoramic radiographs taken in a dental school. J Contemp Dent Pract 2003; 4: 24–34

[5] Rushton MN, Rushton VE, Worthington HV. The value of a quality improvement programme for panoramic radiography: a cluster randomised controlled trial. J Dent 2013; 41: 328–335

[6] Truhlar RS, Morris HF, Ochi S. A review of panoramic radiography and its potential use in implant dentistry. Implant Dent 1993; 2: 122–130

[7] Kim YK, Park JY, Kim SG, Kim JS, Kim JD. Magnification rate of digital panoramic radiographs and its effectiveness for pre-operative assessment of dental implants. Dentomaxillofac Radiol 2011; 40: 76–83

[8] Razi T, Moslemzade SH, Razi S. Comparison of linear dimensions and angular measurements on panoramic images taken with two machines. J Dent Res Dent Clin Dent Prospect 2009; 3: 7–10

[9] Fatahi HR, Babouei EA. Evaluation of the precision of panoramic radiography in dimensional measurements and mandibular steepness in relation to lateral cephalometry. J Mashhad Dental School 2007; 31: 223–230

[10] Van Elslande DC, Russett SJ, Major PW, Flores-Mir C. Mandibular asymmetry diagnosis with panoramic imaging. Am J Orthod Dentofacial Orthop 2008; 134: 183–192

[11] White SC, Pharoah MJ. Intraoral radiographic examinations. In: Oral Radiology: Principles and Interpretation. 6th ed. St. Louis, MO: Mosby; 2009:109–151

[12] Whaites E, Drage N. Periapical radiography. In: Essentials of Dental Radiography and Radiology. 5th ed. Edinburgh: Churchill Livingstone; 2013:85–118

[13] Newman ME, Friedman S. Extraoral radiographic technique: an alternative approach. J Endod 2003; 29: 419–421

[14] Chen CH, Lin SH, Chiu HL, Lin YJ, Chen YK, Lin LM. An aiming device for an extraoral radiographic technique. J Endod 2007; 33: 758–760

[15] Kumar R, Khambete N, Priya E. Extraoral periapical radiography: an alternative approach to intraoral periapical radiography. Imaging Sci Dent 2011; 41: 161–165

[16] Miracle AC, Mukherji SK. Conebeam CT of the head and neck, part 1: physical principles. AJNR Am J Neuroradiol 2009; 30: 1088–1095

[17] Miracle AC, Mukherji SK. Conebeam CT of the head and neck, part 2: clinical applications. AJNR Am J Neuroradiol 2009; 30: 1285–1292

[18] Hodez C, Griffaton-Taillandier C, Bensimon I. Cone-beam imaging: applications in ENT. Eur Ann Otorhinolaryngol Head Neck Dis 2011; 128: 65–78

[19] Campbell PD Jr, Zinreich SJ, Aygun N. Imaging of the paranasal sinuses and in-office CT. Otolaryngol Clin North Am 2009; 42: 753–764, vii

[20] Patel S. New dimensions in endodontic imaging: Part 2. Cone beam computed tomography. Int Endod J 2009; 42: 463–475

[21] Loubele M, Bogaerts R, Van Dijck E et al. Comparison between effective radiation dose of CBCT and MSCT scanners for dentomaxillofacial applications. Eur J Radiol 2009; 71: 461–468

[22] Jeong DK, Lee SC, Huh KH et al. Comparison of effective dose for imaging of mandible between multi-detector CT and cone-beam CT. Imaging Sci Dent 2012; 42: 65–70

[23] Hofmann E, Schmid M, Lell M, Hirschfelder U. Cone beam computed tomography and low-dose multislice computed tomography in orthodontics and dentistry: a comparative evaluation on image quality and radiation exposure. J Orofac Orthop 2014; 75: 384–398

[24] Pauwels R, Beinsberger J, Stamatakis H et al. SEDENTEXCT Project Consortium. Comparison of spatial and contrast resolution for cone-beam computed tomography scanners. Oral Surg Oral Med Oral Pathol Oral Radiol 2012; 114: 127–135

[25] Baba R, Ueda K, Okabe M. Using a flat-panel detector in high resolution cone beam CT for dental imaging. Dentomaxillofac Radiol 2004; 33: 285–290

[26] Pauwels R, Stamatakis H, Bosmans H et al. SEDENTEXCT Project Consortium. Quantification of metal artifacts on cone beam computed tomography images. Clin Oral Implants Res 2013; 24 Suppl A100: 94–99

[27] Brook I. Sinusitis of odontogenic origin. Otolaryngol Head Neck Surg 2006; 135: 349–355

[28] Patel NA, Ferguson BJ. Odontogenic sinusitis: an ancient but underappreciated cause of maxillary sinusitis. Curr Opin Otolaryngol Head Neck Surg 2012; 20: 24–28

[29] Kretzschmar DP, Kretzschmar JL. Rhinosinusitis: review from a dental perspective. Oral Surg Oral Med Oral Pathol Oral Radiol Endod 2003; 96: 128–135

[30] Saibene AM, Pipolo GC, Lozza P et al. Redefining boundaries in odontogenic sinusitis: a retrospective evaluation of extramaxillary involvement in 315 patients. Int Forum Allergy Rhinol 2014; 4: 1020–1023

[31] Lechien JR, Filleul O, Costa de Araujo P, Hsieh JW, Chantrain G, Saussez S. Chronic maxillary rhinosinusitis of dental origin: a systematic review of 674 patient cases. Int J Otolaryngol 2014; 2014: 465173

[32] Costa F, Emanuelli E, Robiony M, Zerman N, Polini F, Politi M. Endoscopic surgical treatment of chronic maxillary sinusitis of dental origin. J Oral Maxillofac Surg 2007; 65: 223–228

[33] Longhini AB, Ferguson BJ. Clinical aspects of odontogenic maxillary sinusitis: a case series. Int Forum Allergy Rhinol 2011; 1: 409–415

[34] Patel S, Dawood A, Ford TP, Whaites E. The potential applications of cone beam computed tomography in the management of endodontic problems. Int Endod J 2007; 40: 818–830

[35] Mengel R, Kruse B, Flores-de-Jacoby L. Digital volume tomography in the diagnosis of peri-implant defects: an in vitro study on native pig mandibles. J Periodontol 2006; 77: 1234–1241

[36] Dave M, Davies J, Wilson R, Palmer R. A comparison of cone beam computed tomography and conventional periapical radiography at detecting peri-implant bone defects. Clin Oral Implants Res 2013; 24: 671–678

[37] Shahbazian M, Vandewoude C, Wyatt J, Jacobs R. Comparative assessment of periapical radiography and CBCT imaging for radiodiagnostics in the posterior maxilla. Odontology 2015;103:97–104

[38] Shiki K, Tanaka T, Kito S et al. The significance of cone beam computed tomography for the visualization of anatomical variations and lesions in the maxillary sinus for patients hoping to have dental implant-supported maxillary restorations in a private dental office in Japan. Head Face Med 2014; 10: 20

[39] Hernando J, Gallego L, Junquera L, Villarreal P. Oroantral communications. A retrospective analysis. Med Oral Patol Oral Cir Bucal 2010; 15: e499–e503

[40] Maillet M, Bowles WR, McClanahan SL, John MT, Ahmad M. Cone-beam computed tomography evaluation of maxillary sinusitis. J Endod 2011; 37: 753–757

[41] Shahbazian M, Jacobs R. Diagnostic value of 2D and 3D imaging in odontogenic maxillary sinusitis: a review of literature. J Oral Rehabil 2012; 39: 294–300

[42] Yadav RK, Chand S, Verma P, Chandra A, Tikku AP, Wadhwani KK. Clinical negligence or endodontic mishaps: A surgeons dilemma. Natl J Maxillofac Surg 2012; 3: 87–90

[43] Raghoebar GM, van Weissenbruch R, Vissink A. Rhino-sinusitis related to endosseous implants extending into the nasal cavity. A case report. Int J Oral Maxillofac Surg 2004; 33: 312–314

[44] Jung JH, Choi BH, Jeong SM, Li J, Lee SH, Lee HJ. A retrospective study of the effects on sinus complications of exposing dental implants to the maxillary sinus cavity. Oral Surg Oral Med Oral Pathol Oral Radiol Endod 2007; 103: 623–625

[45] Manor Y, Mardinger O, Bietlitum I, Nashef A, Nissan J, Chaushu G. Late signs and symptoms of maxillary sinusitis after sinus augmentation. Oral Surg Oral Med Oral Pathol Oral Radiol Endod 2010; 110: e1–e4

[46] Mensi M, Piccioni M, Marsili F, Nicolai P, Sapelli PL, Latronico N. Risk of maxillary fungus ball in patients with endodontic treatment on maxillary teeth: a case-control study. Oral Surg Oral Med Oral Pathol Oral Radiol Endod 2007; 103: 433–436

[47] Park GY, Kim HY, Min JY, Dhong HJ, Chung SK. Endodontic treatment: a significant risk factor for the development of maxillary fungal ball. Clin Exp Otorhinolaryngol 2010; 3: 136–140

[48] Nicolai P, Lombardi D, Tomenzoli D et al. Fungus ball of the paranasal sinuses: experience in 160 patients treated with endoscopic surgery. Laryngoscope 2009; 119: 2275–2279

[49] Yoon JH, Na DG, Byun HS, Koh YH, Chung SK, Dong HJ. Calcification in chronic maxillary sinusitis: comparison of CT findings with histopathologic results. AJNR Am J Neuroradiol 1999; 20: 571–574

[50] Koymen R, Gocmen-Mas N, Karacayli U, Ortakoglu K, Ozen T, Yazici AC. Anatomic evaluation of maxillary sinus septa: surgery and radiology. Clin Anat 2009; 22: 563–570

[51] Mardinger O, Manor I, Mijiritsky E, Hirshberg A. Maxillary sinus augmentation in the presence of antral pseudocyst: a clinical approach. Oral Surg Oral Med Oral Pathol Oral Radiol Endod 2007; 103: 180–184

[52] Tanaka R, Hayashi T. Ohshima H, Ida-Yonemochi H, Kenmotsu S, Ike M. CT anatomy of the anterior superior alveolar nerve canal: a macroscopic and microscopic study. Oral Radiol 2011; 27: 93–97

[53] Ilgüy D, Ilgüy M, Dolekoglu S, Fisekcioglu E. Evaluation of the posterior superior alveolar artery and the maxillary sinus with CBCT. Braz Oral Res 2013; 27: 431–437

Chapter 3

Paranasal Sinuses: Complications following Dental Pathologies or Treatments

3 Paranasal Sinuses: Complications following Dental Pathologies or Treatments

Matteo Chiapasco, Alberto Maria Saibene, Marco Zaniboni, Pierpaolo Racco, Aldo Bruno Giannì

Contents Overview

The aim of this chapter is to describe the main causes of sinonasal pathologies determined by odontogenic conditions or by complications occurring during or after dental treatments. These include: infection or necrosis of the maxillary teeth (both primary and secondary to incomplete or improper endodontic treatment); infection around oral implants placed in the maxilla with secondary involvement of the sinonasal cavities; penetration or displacement of oral implants into the nasal and paranasal cavities; and infection following sinus grafting procedures to allow implant placement in the atrophic lateral-posterior maxilla. A classification is provided at the beginning of the chapter along with a flow chart for everyday practice.

3.1 Introduction: Classification

Odontogenic sinusitis has traditionally been related to dental conditions such as periodontal pathologies, pulpitis, or infection of odontogenic cysts. However, the great expansion in the use of oral implants in the last three decades, as well as regenerative procedures for bone augmentation in the posterior maxilla (including bone grafting of the maxillary sinus, the so-called sinus lift), has led to an increase in paranasal sinus involvement, as a consequence of complications of these procedures (penetration/migration of dental implants and/or grafting materials into the maxillary sinus). It is generally assumed that approximately 30% of maxillary sinus infections can be ascribed to an odontogenic cause.[1]

Otolaryngologists, as well as oral and maxillofacial surgeons, are therefore frequently involved in the management of sinonasal inflammatory or infectious conditions deriving from: (1) the absence of treatment or the improper management of infections involving the lateral-posterior dentition of the maxilla; and (2) the placement of implants and reconstructive procedures in the edentulous posterior maxilla.

For this reason, newer classification systems have attempted to integrate classic odontogenic sinusitis and other frequent sinonasal conditions not directly related to the teeth or to other types of sinusitis, such as implant-related and sinus augmentation-related adverse events, into the definition of *sinonasal complications of dental disease or treatment* (SCDDT).

To allow the creation of standardized treatment protocols and encourage cooperation among clinicians of different specialties, we have proposed an SCDDT classification (▶ Table 3.1). According to their etiology, SCDDT are classified in three groups: (1) complications following bone augmentation procedures in the edentulous atrophic posterior maxilla; (2) implant-related complications; and (3) dental diseases and complications of dental treatments. Each group has been divided into different classes according to the initial clinical situation and the proposed treatment modalities. It is worth noting that individual patients may present different clinical situations that are included in different classes. To classify the most complex cases, a ranking system has been devised: the ranking system mirrors the disruption of sinonasal homeostasis, which is markedly more extensive in group I patients, with a gradual reduction toward group III, class 3b. ▶ Table 3.1 summarizes the groups and classes.

3.2 Classic Odontogenic Sinusitis (Group III, Classes 3a, 3b)

3.2.1 Introduction

The roots of the upper teeth are embedded in the maxillary alveolar crest, which rises from the horizontal plate of the palatine bone on the oral side and from the base of the maxillary bone on the buccal side. In the frontal area of the maxilla (premaxilla), the radicular apices of the incisors, because of the dimension and position of their roots, may be in close proximity to the floor of the nasal cavity, while in the lateral-posterior areas of the maxilla, the radicular apices of the premolars and molars may

Table 3.1 Classification of SCDDT patients

Groups	I	Complications related to maxillary sinus grafting
	II	Complications related to oral implants
	III	Complications related to dental pathologies and treatments
Classes	1a	Sinusitis following sinus grafting
	2a	Sinusitis with peri-implantitis and OAC
	2b	Sinusitis following implant displacement with OAC
	2c	Sinusitis following implant displacement
	2d	Implant displacement without sinusitis
	3a	Odontogenic sinusitis with OAC
	3b	Odontogenic sinusitis

Abbreviations: OAC, oroantral communication; SCDDT, sinonasal complications of dental disease or treatment.

have a similar spatial relationship with the maxillary sinuses. The apices of the premolar and molar teeth are, in fact, separated from the floor of the sinus by a thin layer of bone and, not infrequently, may even protrude into the floor of the sinus when the roots are long or the sinus is enlarged.

This anatomical contiguity increases the likelihood that a pathological process affecting the dental pulp of premolar and molar teeth (typically, necrosis followed by infection) or a periodontal infection reaching the apices of these teeth will be conveyed to the maxillary sinus. In addition, improper endodontic treatment of these teeth may leave bacteria or necrotic material in (or even push them into) the sinus, leading to the clinical condition termed *odontogenic sinusitis*. When odontogenic sinusitis occurs, regardless of the etiology, common endoscopic findings are a purulent discharge coming from the middle meatus and/or anteriorization of the uncinate process caused by the pressure of the purulent content of the sinus.

3.2.2 Clinical Scenarios

Dental Pathologies with Secondary Involvement of the Maxillary Sinus

This group of conditions includes infectious pathologies originating from: (1) pulpal necrosis caused by migration of bacteria from the oral cavity into the pulpal spaces of a tooth (generally premolar and molar teeth or, more rarely, canines) affected by deep caries or fracture of the crown/root; (2) pulpal necrosis of a tooth with no crown/root caries or fracture; and (3) infection of an odontogenic cyst.

When a carious process is left untreated, the destructive action of the bacteria involved in the pathological process leads to the dissolution of large portions of dental substance, finally involving the roof of the pulp chamber. When this happens, the pulpal tissues are exposed not only to the bacteria (and their toxins) that originally led to the carious process, but also to bacteria and toxins that are present in the oral cavity and fluids. A similar scenario occurs in the case of crown fractures involving both the enamel layer and the underlying dentine layer: the pulp chamber is violated and the pulp exposed.

In these circumstances, the action of the microorganisms leads to the necrosis of the vital pulp: bacteria spread into the tissues and dentinal tubules, eliciting a response from the immune system. Neutrophil granulocytes migrate into the area by chemotaxis and start to phagocytose bacteria. Once ingested, bacteria are isolated in membrane-bound phagosomes and killed by an aerobic mechanism that leads to the formation of intracellular oxygen-derived free radicals ("respiratory burst") in the initial phase, and then by an anaerobic mechanism in which the phagosomes fuse with the neutrophil's own intracellular primary and secondary granules containing lytic enzymes that digest the microbes.[2] The neutrophils are mobilized to eliminate pathogens, but they can also cause severe damage to host tissues. The enzymes contained in their granules (neutral proteinases, myeloperoxidase, lysosomes, cationic proteins, matrix metalloproteinases), once released, degrade the structural elements of cells, tissues, and the extracellular matrix, because they do not discriminate between pathogens and host tissues.

For this reason, the accumulation of neutrophils is the first cause of pulpal tissue dissolution during the first (acute) phase of the infection.[3] This process then spreads apically along the root canals until it reaches the apical region of the tooth and is conveyed through the apical foramen into the periapical region, involving the periodontal ligament and periradicular bone. The most prominent bacterial groups detectable in the apical 5 mm of infected root canals in teeth with pulpal exposure are *Actinomyces, Lactobacillus*, black-pigmented *Bacteroides, Peptostreptococcus*, nonpigmented *Bacteroides, Veillonella, Enterococcus faecalis, Fusobacterium nucleatum*, and *Streptococcus mutans*; 68% of the bacterial population is composed of strict anaerobes.[4] Migration of the infectious process out of the apex (in the case of roots protruding into the lumen of the maxillary sinus) or lysis of the thin layer of bone separating the tip of the root from the floor of the sinus leads to the diffusion of infectious and necrotic material into the maxillary sinus, ultimately resulting in an odontogenic sinusitis (▶ Fig. 3.1).

In the second type of pathology seen in Group III, the pathological process is very similar; the only, albeit significant, difference is that necrosis of the pulpal tissues occurs in the absence of caries or crown fractures. However, the application of advanced laboratory techniques for the detection and isolation of anaerobes has demonstrated that the root canal flora of teeth with clinically intact crowns, but suffering from pulpal necrosis and periapical reactions, is largely composed of obligate anaerobes (>90%) belonging to the genera *Fusobacterium, Porphyromonas, Prevotella, Eubacterium*, and *Peptostreptococcus*.[5] The pulpal necrosis may therefore be the result of an alteration in the microbial interactions influencing the ecology of the endodontic flora. These interactions include either positive (synergic) or negative associations that can cause alterations in the environment of the entire root canal system (e.g., presence and concentration of nutrients and gases). For example, it has been demonstrated that in the early stages of pulpal infection facultative anaerobes are predominant in the microflora[6] and they use the available oxygen for their metabolic processes, leading to a drop in the intrapulpal partial pressure of oxygen.[7] In an environment with low levels of oxygen, the growth of obligate anaerobes is favored and the result is the multiplication of these bacteria inside the tooth.[6] Moreover, the by-products or end products of the metabolic processes of some families of bacteria may act as nutrients for other types of microorganisms.[8,9] Within this virtually closed system, all of these variables may

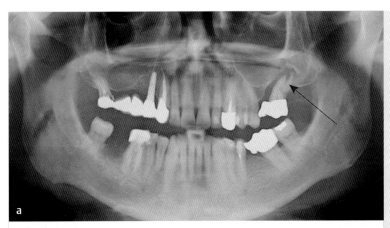

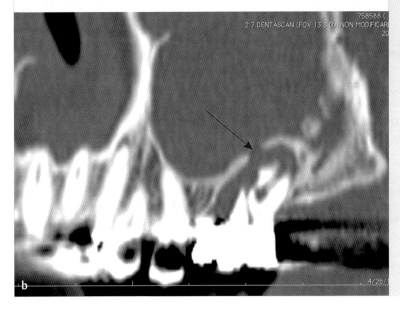

Fig. 3.1 (a, b) Odontogenic maxillary sinusitis caused by endodontic and periodontal infection involving the upper left second molar (*arrow*). The original infection eroded the floor of the sinus (*arrow*) and spread into the lumen.

lead to significant variations in the bacterial composition inside the root canal spaces.

On the other hand, external factors that can lead to pulpal necrosis may be physical (e.g., trauma, heat) or chemical (e.g., acids). A physical trauma can sever the fine blood vessels and nerve fibers that enter the root canal system through the apical foramen, leaving the tooth without a blood supply and thus causing necrosis of the pulpal tissues. Thermal injury, for example by hot ingested substances or inadequate cooling of burs during tooth preparation, may result in irreversible damage to the structure of the pulpal tissues and subsequent necrosis of the pulp. Finally, chemicals used as etchants in adhesive procedures (e.g., application of veneers, composite restorations) or as a base under restorations may alter the characteristics of the dentin (by widening the openings of dentinal tubules, increasing dentin permeability, and enhancing bacterial penetration of the dentin) and of the endodontic environment and cause damage to the pulpal tissues that may be irreversible and lead to pulpal necrosis. The end result, as described in the previous scenario, is the migration of the by-products of pulpal necrosis through the root canal system and out of the apex. When these materials spread into the lumen of the maxillary sinus (because the roots of the tooth protrude through the floor of the sinus or because these materials cause the lysis of the periapical bone and the floor of the sinus) an odontogenic sinusitis occurs.

Finally, in the third type of pathology associated with group III, an odontogenic cyst originating from a periapical granuloma as a consequence of tooth necrosis may be responsible for an odontogenic sinusitis. Odontogenic (periapical) cysts generally have a slow expansion pattern and can develop for months or even years without any signs or symptoms. They originate from a periapical granuloma that enlarges progressively and provides itself with an epithelial or connective tissue wall separating the lesion from the surrounding bone and containing the infectious and/or necrotic material that supports its expansion.

The mechanism behind the growth of odontogenic cysts is still under debate, and two different hypotheses share the support of the scientific community: the hydrostatic theory[10] and the prostaglandin theory.[11] According to the hydrostatic theory, the degeneration of cells inside the cyst causes an accumulation of organic remains (e.g., proteins, cholesterol crystals, cytoplasmic bodies), leading to an increase in the osmotic pressure inside the original focus; this causes liquids from the surrounding tissues to migrate into the cyst through its semipermeable membrane, thus increasing the inner hydrostatic pressure. The pressure exerted by the intracystic fluids on the surrounding bone may trigger an osteoclastic activation, which in turn initiates the osteolytic process.

On the other hand, according to the prostaglandin theory, the cyst wall may be able to produce and release substances such as prostaglandins and prostacyclins from either its epithelial or its connective tissue components, and these are able to activate osteoclast pools with subsequent perilesional bone resorption. Whatever the mechanism of the growth of the cyst, and both the processes described are likely to be involved, the expansion continues until the cortical wall of the surrounding bone has been consumed and, with the formation of a fistula (intraoral or extraoral), the intracystic fluid can drain spontaneously. When the drainage occurs through an intraoral or cutaneous fistula (typically in the malar region for upper posterior teeth) the clinician and even the patient can easily recognize that an infectious process is ongoing. When, on the other hand, the drainage occurs inside the maxillary sinus it may go unnoticed, and the infectious material may cause an odontogenic sinusitis (▶ Fig. 3.2).

Complications of Dental Treatments with Secondary Involvement of the Maxillary Sinus

Maxillary sinus infection may also be a consequence of improper treatment of premolars and molars (and, more rarely, canines). These treatments may include the reconstruction of teeth affected by severe decay (e.g., deep caries), endodontic therapies, or tooth extractions.

As far as reconstruction of severely compromised teeth are concerned, the causes of puplar necrosis may be: (1) previous migration of bacteria into the dental pulp through the dentinal tubules present in the thin layer of residual dentin above the pulp chamber; (2) chemical insult from the materials (resins) used for adhesive restoration of the tooth; (3) restorations lacking adequate marginal seal, leading to marginal leakage of contaminated oral fluids and migration of bacteria inside the dentinal tubules up to the pulp chamber; (4) failure of procedures such as direct or indirect capping of the exposed dental pulp; (5) erroneous restoration of teeth that, following a correct diagnostic examination, should have been treated with endodontic therapy prior to reconstruction of the crown.[12]

All of these possible causes of pulpal necrosis following dental restoration may lead to the same sequelae described in the previous section for noniatrogenic damage to the dental pulp, with migration of the by-products of the necrotic process through the apical foramen, from where they can spread either directly (if the root protrudes through the floor of the maxillary sinus) or indirectly (when the necrotic/infectious material causes lysis of the thin layer of bone separating the root from the floor of the sinus) into the lumen of the maxillary sinus and lead to infection.

In the case of endodontic treatment, complete elimination of organic materials from, and thorough disinfection of, the root canal system, and finally competent three-dimensional obturation of all spaces using adequate filling materials are all necessary to avoid sinusitis, in particular when the apices of the roots are very close to the sinusal floor or protrude into it. In order to perform a correct endodontic treatment, all the procedures must be carried out after adequate isolation of the working field with a sheet of rubber dental dam. This essential

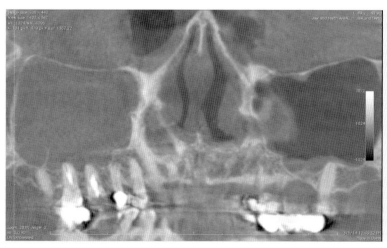

Fig. 3.2 An odontogenic cyst, originating from endodontically treated upper right molars, which has expanded into the maxillary sinus with secondary diffusion of the infectious content into the lumen of the sinus.

precaution prevents the migration of contaminated oral fluids into the exposed pulpal spaces, both in the first phase of the treatment (when the pulp chamber is opened with a bur mounted on a handpiece and the necrotic tissues are removed from the root canal system) and in the second phase of the treatment (when the root canal system is correctly shaped, disinfected, and obturated). If the working field is not properly isolated with the rubber dam, there can never be certainty that the root canal system is not contaminated by bacteria, even if all the procedures are carried out properly. If this occurs, signs of necrosis or infection may become radiographically visible in the periapical/periradicular bone months after the completion of the treatment and even if the filling of the root canals appears to be complete.[12]

Another possible cause of maxillary sinusitis related to endodontic treatment is the erroneous modification of the natural anatomy of the most apical portion of the root canal during the shaping maneuvers carried out with manual and/or rotary instruments. If the length and anatomy of the root canal are not assessed with precision, or if the size of the file to be used for the shaping is not chosen with care, the naturally retentive form of the apical extremity of the root canal (the "anatomical apex") may be altered. When this occurs, apical retention is eliminated and the necrotic/infected pulpal tissue remnants or the endodontic materials used in the course of the treatment can be pushed out of the apex and penetrate the maxillary sinus.[12]

In addition, improper use of disinfectants for the elimination of bacteria and organic tissues may be followed by a sinus reaction. Irrigation with disinfectants in the course of endodontic treatment should be carried out with specifically designed needles, in which the terminal hole is not located on top of the tip but on the side of it, to allow the irrigant solutions to flow in the coronal direction and not toward the apex. Moreover, the pressure applied to the piston of the syringe should not be excessive, and the needle should be positioned inside the root canal in such a way that it is not stuck but can be moved freely, leaving enough room for the liquids to flow out of the coronal opening of the canal. If these principles are not followed, the pressure of the fluids inside the root canal may exceed the resistance offered by the natural form of the anatomical apex, and the disinfectants can flow out of the apex and into the periapical bone. These substances may be either basic (e.g., sodium chloride) or acidic (e.g., hydrogen peroxide) and, when flowing out of the apex, can damage the periapical tissues (periodontal ligament, bone). Drainage into the lumen of the sinus also damages Schneider's membrane and evokes an acute inflammatory response.[12]

Similarly, the materials used to fill the cleaned and shaped root canal system (cements and gutta percha,

both of which are carried inside the canals in a fluid form) can flow out of the apex and into the periapical bone or sinusal cavity. Cements may produce an effect similar to that described for irrigants, while gutta percha solidifies and may evoke foreign body–type reactions[12] (▶ Fig. 3.3) or may even facilitate extramucosal mycosis, as described in Chapter 4 (p. 66).

Complications of tooth extraction procedures occur when incautious operative maneuvers result in the dislocation into the maxillary sinus of a root fragment, a root, or even the entire tooth (particularly in the case of roots already penetrating into the sinus or impacted teeth). Displacement into the maxillary sinus may lead to either: (1) spontaneous expulsion of root fragments or roots/teeth through the ostium (as a result of mucociliary activity) into the nasal cavity and, from there, either out of the nostrils or down into the pharynx; or (2) the persistence of the root/tooth in the maxillary sinus.

Spontaneous expulsion may occur in the case of a relatively small fragment and a patent and relatively large ostium, while it is less likely to happen when the fragment is large, of unfavorable shape, or when the ostium is partially or completely obstructed. If the root fragment is expelled from the maxillary sinus into the nasal cavity, it may migrate into the trachea and the bronchial system, with the risk of developing a lung infection.

The persistence of a root or a tooth in the sinus (as with oral implants displaced into the sinus) can be followed either by the absence of symptoms and signs of infection (apart from a sinus mucosal reaction and thickening, but without significant infection/sinusitis), or by an acute or chronic maxillary sinusitis. The latter may spread to other paranasal sinuses, potentially leading to major complications such as the involvement of the orbital cavity (with a risk of orbital cellulitis and damage to the optic nerve), or the intracranial cavity (with a risk of meningitis and/or brain abscesses), as has also been described in patients with other foreign bodies displaced into the maxillary sinus or in patients with odontogenic sinusitis originating from infected dental roots and improper endodontic treatment[13–15] (▶ Fig. 3.4).

Tooth extraction maneuvers may also produce *oroantral communications* (OAC). This complication may be inevitable when one or more roots protrude into the sinus floor, but it may also be the result of an improper extraction procedure, leading to fracture of the floor of the sinus and the creation of an oroantral communication (▶ Fig. 3.5). Irrespective of the cause, the communication must be promptly closed with appropriate techniques (generally with a local mucosal flap), to avoid the formation of an oroantral fistula that would maintain a continuous migration of bacteria from the oral cavity into the sinus and vice versa, with the potential development of sinusitis.

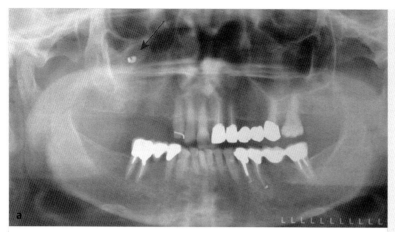

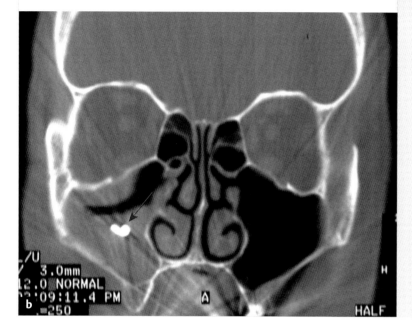

Fig. 3.3 (**a, b**) Endodontic material (*arrow*) previously used to treat a necrotic molar tooth (which was then extracted) has dispersed into the maxillary sinus. A foreign body reaction has developed into an odontogenic sinusitis.

3.3 Complications following the Use of Oral Implants in the Upper Jaw (Infection/Displacement) (Group II, Classes 2a, 2b, 2c, 2d)

3.3.1 Introduction

The rehabilitation of partially or totally edentulous patients with implant-supported prostheses has become common practice in recent decades, with reliable long-term results. Natural tooth roots can be replaced by oral implants, on which it is possible to construct single or multiple prosthetic crowns.

A fundamental prerequisite for long-term survival of oral implants is osseointegration of the implant into the bone. This well-studied process is characterized by the formation of a functional ankylosis of the implant into the bone in order to develop the maximum direct bone-to-implant contact. Although many types of implants have been introduced into the market in the last four decades (blade implants, subperiosteal implants, etc.), a large body of literature, including both animal and clinical studies, has demonstrated the process of osseointegration only for root-form titanium implants.[16-19]

The second important factor for successful osseointegration is the presence of an adequate volume of residual bone in terms of height and width of the alveolar crest, to allow complete embedding of the whole implant surface into the bone.

However, edentulous alveolar ridges may be unfavorable for implant placement. The loss of teeth is always followed by a progressive and three-dimensional resorption of the alveolar bone, which follows relatively

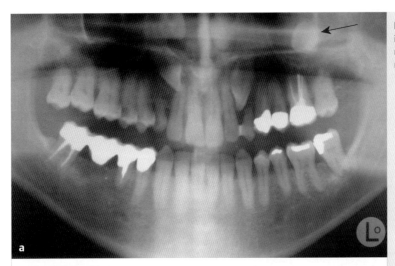

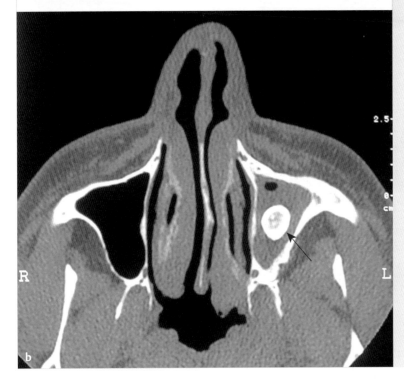

Fig. 3.4 (a, b) Odontogenic sinusitis following displacement of an upper left third molar (*arrow*) as a result of using incorrect maneuvers during an extraction.

predictable patterns, albeit very variable between patients[20]; this may render implant placement difficult or impossible. Of the different tooth-bearing areas of the mandible and the maxilla, the edentulous lateral-posterior maxilla is one of the most challenging, because bone resorption is often associated with maxillary sinus expansion, thus leading to a further reduction of the available bone. The re-creation of an adequate bone volume in the anterior and/or lateral-posterior maxilla through bone augmentation procedures such as bone grafts, guided bone regeneration, and elevation and grafting of the floor of the maxillary sinus (the so-called sinus lift) to host implants of

adequate dimensions and in the proper position represents the ideal solution.[21-24]

However, due to inexperience or incorrect planning, it is not unusual for attempts to be made to place implants in reduced residual bone. Although not systematically described in the literature, several complications have been reported relating to loss or absence of osseointegration, or penetration or displacement of implants into the nasal cavity or maxillary sinus. Both partial penetration and complete displacement of implants may remain clinically silent or may be followed by a foreign body reaction, leading to infection of the maxillary sinus. If not properly treated, maxillary sinus infection may

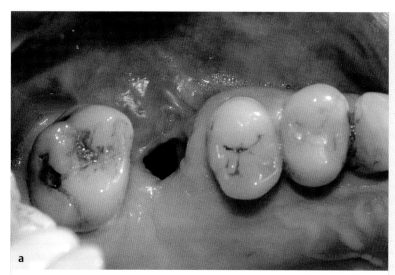

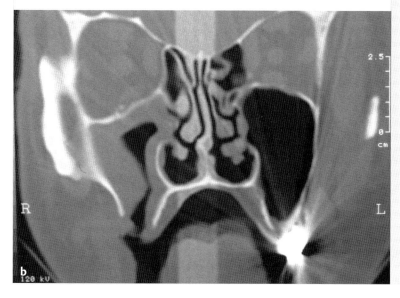

Fig. 3.5 (a) Clinical and (b) radiographic view of an oroantral communication following extraction of the upper right first molar, with development of maxillary sinusitis.

involve other paranasal sinuses (ethmoid, frontal, and sphenoid sinuses) or, even worse, may spread to the orbital cavity or the cranial cavity, with potentially severe complications, as already described for displacement of dental roots into the maxillary sinus.[13–15,25] The aim of this section is to describe the clinical scenarios that may develop as a result of penetration or displacement of implants into the maxillary sinus.

3.3.2 Clinical Scenarios

Partial Penetration of an Implant into the Maxillary Sinus without Peri-implant Infection

The partial penetration of an implant into the maxillary sinus is not always followed by complications. As long

ago as 1984, Brånemark et al[26] demonstrated that implants penetrating 2 to 3 mm into the maxillary sinus did not cause sinus infection in the majority of patients. The tip of the implant that had torn Schneider's membrane was probably covered after several weeks or months by newly formed sinus membrane epithelium. It is worth noting, however, that the observations reported by Brånemark et al[26] were related to the so-called machined-surface implants. The surface of these implants (nowadays more rarely used) presents a smooth surface that is potentially less prone to bacterial contamination. The majority of modern implants are characterized by varying degrees of micro-roughness, which has been introduced to increase the area of bone-to-implant contact, thereby improving osseointegration. These surfaces, however, may potentially be more prone to bacterial contamination and therefore expose the patient to a higher risk of sinus infection. Periodic clinical and radiographic check-ups are therefore indicated, because an infection can develop also time after the initial penetration of the implant into the maxillary sinus (▶ Fig. 3.6).

Partial Penetration of an Implant into the Maxillary Sinus with Infection (Class 2a)

As in any other part of the tooth-bearing area, the implant surface is exposed to a low risk of bacterial contamination, involving the implant surface and the surrounding hard and soft tissues, termed *peri-implantitis*. It is well known that the oral cavity is populated by many types of bacteria; however, in healthy patients with adequate levels of oral hygiene, no periodontal disease in the surrounding dentition, and an adequate "seal" of peri-implant soft tissues no infection develops, as with

the natural teeth. If this peri-implant seal is lost and significant quantities of bacteria accumulate, particularly in the absence of an adequate level of oral hygiene, bacteria may penetrate at different levels around the implant, causing acute or chronic infection. Peri-implantitis may involve only the most coronal part of the implant (the part closest to the alveolar crest and the oral mucosa) or may involve the more apical part of the implant. If this part of the implant has already penetrated the maxillary sinus floor, it is likely that infection will diffuse into the sinus and potentially involve other paranasal cavities, the orbit, and, although very rarely, the cranial fossae, as described in Section 3.2.2 (p. 41) on the complications following improper treatment of teeth (▶ Fig. 3.7).

Whenever the peri-implant infection involves the whole surface of the implant, the latter may lose osseointegration and become mobile. Some old-style fibrous

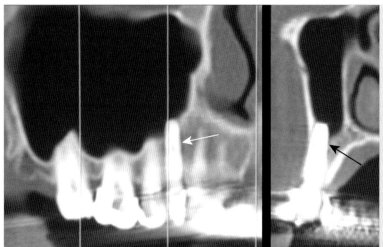

Fig. 3.6 CT scans showing an osseointegrated implant protruding into the maxillary sinus (*arrow*) without signs of sinusitis.

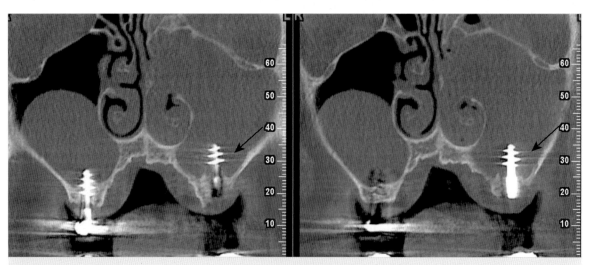

Fig. 3.7 CT scans showing an implant protruding into the left maxillary sinus (*arrow*), with infectious involvement of the maxillary sinus and ethmoidal cells.

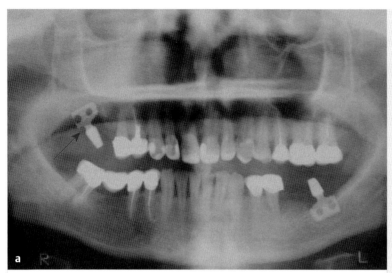

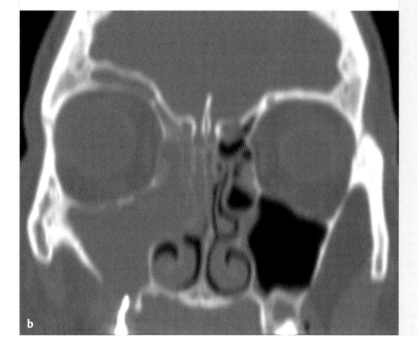

Fig. 3.8 **(a)** A Linkow blade–type implant displaced into the maxillary sinus (*arrow*) following loss of integration and destruction of the alveolar bone by infection. **(b)** The CT scan shows the diffusion of the infectious process to the maxillary sinus, the ethmoidal cells, and the frontal sinus.

integrated implants, such as the Linkow blades, are more prone to this complication (▸ Fig. 3.8).

Finally, another type of implant, the so-called subperiosteal implant, may become infected. When this happens, infection may first involve the soft tissues surrounding the maxillary bone (with potential evolution toward cellulitis or necrotizing fasciitis) and then lead to infection or resorption of the bone. This latter event is generally followed by implant mobility and penetration

of the implant into the sinus with large-scale destruction of the bony walls, leading to oroantral communications (▸ Fig. 3.9).

Displacement of an Implant into the Maxillary Sinus (Classes 2b, 2c, 2d)

Due to inexperience, incorrect planning, or intraoperative mistakes, typically in patients with poor quality and

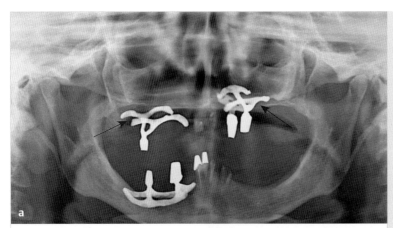

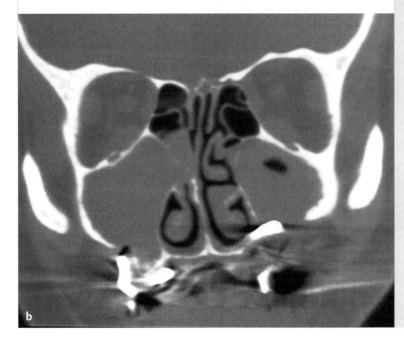

Fig. 3.9 (a) Infection around subperiosteal implants (*arrows*) causing complete destruction of the alveolar ridge with subsequent penetration of the implants into the maxillary sinus. **(b)** The CT scan clearly shows that both maxillary sinuses and some ethmoidal cells are involved in the infectious process.

quantity of residual alveolar bone in the lateral-posterior maxilla, an oral implant may be completely displaced into the maxillary sinus during the surgical procedure or may migrate into the sinus after surgery.[13,25,27]

Displaced implants act as foreign bodies and may lead to different clinical situations: (1) persistence of the implant in the sinus with no inflammatory or infectious reaction (class 2d); (2) spontaneous expulsion of the implant through the maxillary ostium into the nasal cavity (particularly in the case of a large ostium, small implant, efficient ciliary movement, and clearance capacity); (3) persistence of the implant in the sinus followed by an inflammatory reaction or sinusitis (classes 2b and 2c).

The first scenario may persist for long periods of time in the absence of symptoms and signs of infection (besides appreciable signs of reaction, frequently some degree of "thickening", of the sinusal mucosa), but may also evolve at any time into either of the other two scenarios (▶ Fig. 3.10).

The second scenario may be followed by spontaneous expulsion of the implant through the nose (▶ Fig. 3.11) or the oral cavity, but may also lead to ingestion of the implant through the pharynx and the esophagus or to penetration into the larynx and trachea, as described previously for dental roots; this latter situation may be followed by lung infection. An expulsed implant may also

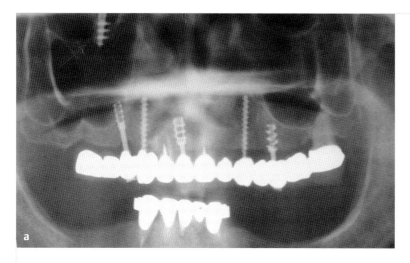

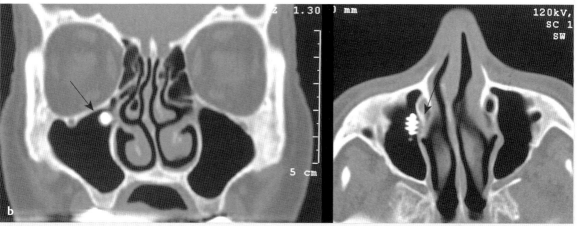

Fig. 3.10 (a) Panoramic radiograph and **(b)** CT scans showing an implant that has migrated into the maxillary sinus (*arrow*) with no significant signs of sinusitis.

migrate toward the ethmoidal cells or the sphenoidal sinus (▶ Fig. 3.12), or even toward the anterior or middle cranial fossae, with potential major complications (meningitis, encephalitis, or brain abscesses, as described previously in Section 3.2.2 [p. 41] for displaced dental roots).

The third scenario is the persistence of an implant in the maxillary sinus followed by a foreign body reaction or infection (class 2c). This encompasses more favorable situations, where there is thickening of the sinusal mucosa with polypoid characteristics, but moderate or no secretion of purulent material, and also less favorable situations where there is acute or chronic sinusitis that may involve only the maxillary sinus, or extend toward other paranasal sinuses, the orbit, or the cranial fossae; the possible clinical developments are as described in the previous sections.

Finally, following intraoperative or postoperative displacement or migration of an implant, an oroantral communication may develop (class 2b), followed by contamination of the sinus by oral bacteria and the

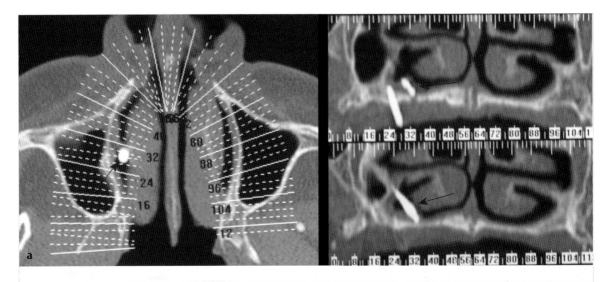

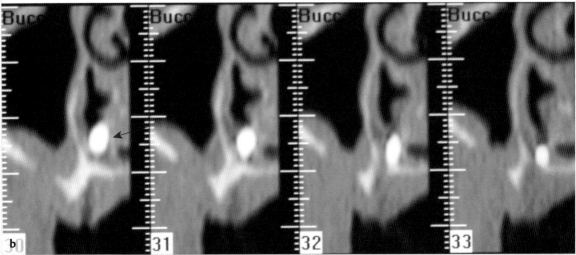

Fig. 3.11 (a) Axial, panoramic, and (b) cross-sectional CT scans showing an implant (*arrow*) originally displaced into the maxillary sinus that spontaneously migrated one week later into the nasal cavity under the inferior turbinate.

development of sinusitis (in addition to problems such as passage of fluids from the oral cavity to the nose through the sinus)[13,25,27] (▶ Fig. 3.13).

3.4 Complications following Maxillary Sinus Grafting Prior to or in Association with Oral Implant Placement (Group I, Class 1a)

As described in the previous section, the prosthetic rehabilitation of partially or totally edentulous patients with osseointegrated oral implants has become a routine treatment with reliable long-term results.[18,19] A prerequisite for the long-term success of oral implants is the presence of an adequate volume of residual alveolar bone in terms of height and width, to host the whole surface of the implant and allow its integration.

However, the loss of teeth is always followed by a progressive, three-dimensional resorption of the alveolar bone.[20] The lateral and posterior edentulous maxilla is one of the most challenging areas for the oral surgeon, because bone resorption is often associated with maxillary sinus expansion, leading to a further reduction of the available bone. In fact, the absence of functional loading during mastication leads to a progressive loss of

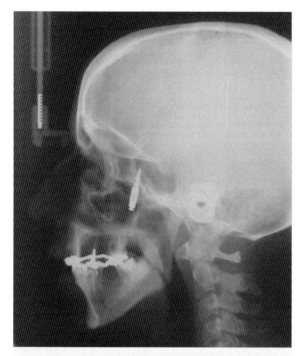

Fig. 3.12 Lateral X-ray showing an implant and its mounting device inside the ostium of the sphenoid sinus. The implant was originally displaced into the maxillary sinus and spontaneously migrated toward the sphenoid.

maxillary bone trophism and favors an expansion of the sinuses, due to the outward air pressure within the maxillary sinus, rendering the placement of oral implants difficult or impossible.[20]

Bone augmentation procedures of the lateral-posterior maxilla have been conceived to overcome these problems and to host implants of adequate dimensions and in the proper position. Two main techniques have been proposed over the years: (1) elevation of the sinus (Schneider's) membrane and grafting of the maxillary sinus floor via a lateral approach; (2) elevation of the sinus membrane through a crestal approach.

3.4.1 Elevation of the Sinus Membrane and Grafting of Maxillary Sinus Floor via a Lateral Approach

This surgical technique was originally introduced to reduce bulky maxillary tuberosities in edentulous patients, thus leading to a reduced interarch distance and difficulties in wearing a removable prosthesis. Briefly, the removed bone was grafted into the floor of the maxillary sinus, after elevation of Schneider's membrane. Three months later, it was therefore possible to reduce the tuberosity without penetrating the maxillary sinus.

The technique currently used to augment the available bone in patients with an expanded maxillary sinus, to

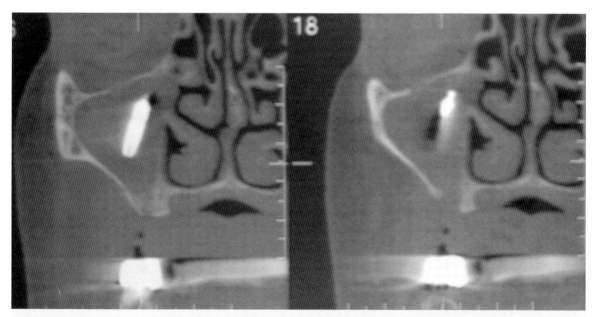

Fig. 3.13 Cross-sectional CT scans showing the migration of an implant and its prosthetic abutment into the maxillary sinus. An oroantral communication is clearly visible, as is the extent of the resulting infection involving the entire lumen of the sinus.

allow the placement of oral implants, was first described by Tatum in 1977[28] and Boyne and James in 1980.[21] It involves the creation of a bony window by eroding the lateral wall of the sinus, followed by the elevation of Schneider's membrane, taking great care not to tear it. The space created is then grafted with autologous bone particles harvested from the anterior ilium.

In the last three decades, this technique has been associated with the modern generation of osseointegrated screw-shaped implants and a variety of grafting materials have been used to obtain the desired bone augmentation. These materials can be classified as autologous grafts (from the same individual), allografts (from the same species), xenografts (from a different species), and alloplastic materials.[24,29,30]

Autologous bone can be used as a block in particulate form: the donor site may be intraoral (mandibular ramus, mandibular symphysis, maxillary tuberosity) or extraoral (iliac crest, calvaria, tibia). The use of bone blocks in sinus lift procedures has been progressively replaced by particulate grafts, as they do not require complex stabilization and show a lower tendency to be resorbed.[31] The advantages of autologous bone are that it is both osteoinductive (directly induces new bone formation by delivering growth factors locally) and osteoconductive (passively acts as a scaffold for new bone formation),[32] it undergoes faster integration compared with other biomaterials, and it allows for a greater amount of vital bone formation in the early stages. Finally, the management of infective complications (if any) can be easier, due to faster revascularization of the graft, which allows for adequate delivery of systemic antibiotics. The disadvantage is the need to harvest autologous bone from a donor site, with increased morbidity and prolongation of surgical times.

Allografts taken from cadavers can be prepared as: (1) freeze-dried bone allograft (FDBA); (2) demineralized freeze-dried bone allograft (DFDBA); or (3) fresh frozen bone allograft (FFBA). These materials have an osteoconductive potential derived from their morphology and they allow stabilization of the clot, promote neoangiogenesis within the graft, and act as a scaffold for the host's new bone cells. However, their osteoinductive properties associated with the presence of bone morphogenetic proteins are still under debate.[32,33]

Xenografts, usually obtained from bovine or equine sources, have only osteoconductive properties and present a rich mineral component, which may guarantee the graft long-term dimensional stability.

The group of alloplastic materials, of natural or synthetic origin, used for grafting includes hydroxyapatites, bioactive glasses, bioceramics, calcium sulfate, calcium phosphate, etc. According to their characteristics, they may have osteoconductive or osteostimulating properties. Osteostimulation means the capacity of the material to stimulate the expression and activity of osteoblasts. Histologically, it is characterized by bone proliferation from the walls of the defect and slow growth within the filled defect and on the surface of the material (centrifugal ossification, distance osteogenesis).[34]

Of these materials, autologous bone and bovine bone mineral xenografts, used alone or in combination, are the best documented materials for sinus grafting procedures. Endosseous implants placed in grafted sinuses have high survival rates (>90% after at least 5 years of follow-up), consistent with those reported for implants placed in native bone.[24,29,30]

Technical Details

The approach to lateral wall of the maxillary sinus is obtained with the elevation of a mucoperiosteal flap on the buccal aspect of the lateral-posterior maxilla. The design of the flap depends on the mesiodistal position of the sinus and the extent of the planned antrostomy (or bony window) and may also vary if bone regeneration or reconstruction of the ridge is needed (in patients with sinus expansion associated with significant horizontal or vertical resorption of the ridge). Once the surgical access is obtained, the limits of the bony window are defined. They vary according to the sinus dimensions, the number of implants to be inserted, and the anatomical features of the sinus (e.g., the presence of Underwood's septa). Generally speaking, the bony window, outlined either with round burs assembled on surgical handpieces or with piezoelectric instruments under irrigation with sterile saline, has an oval shape. The inferior margin is located a few millimeters cranial to the sinus floor, while the mesial limit is usually close to the anterior recess of the maxillary sinus, to facilitate the elevation of Schneider's membrane. The distal limit is related to the extent of the edentulous area, while the upper limit is dictated by the vertical bone gain required. As the healing process leading to the integration of the graft starts from the bone walls, maximum bone-to-graft contact creates the ideal conditions for improving graft stability and blood supply.[35] It is also important to extend the membrane elevation to the medial aspect of the sinus wall: this allows the graft to be in contact with the medial wall of the sinus, thereby leading to a greater blood supply and stability. Moreover, the new floor of the maxillary sinus will not present recesses with acute angles that may interfere with the physiological clearance and drainage of

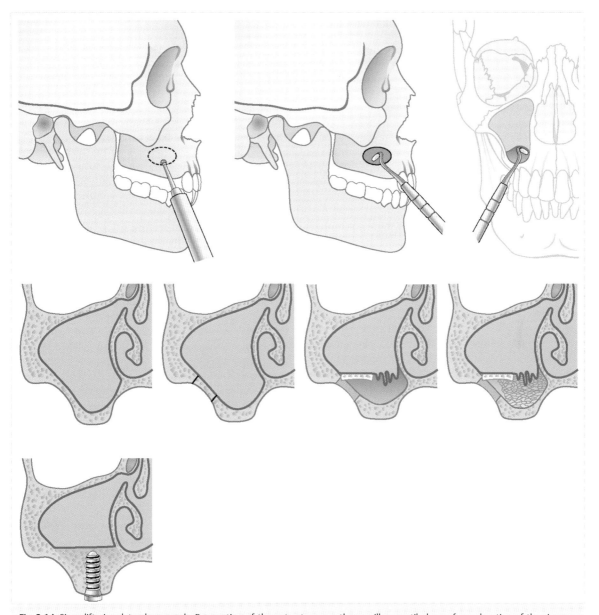

Fig. 3.14 Sinus lift via a lateral approach. Preparation of the antrostomy on the maxillary vestibular surface, elevation of the sinus membrane, placement and consolidation of the grafting material, and insertion of an implant in the second stage.

maxillary sinus secretions toward the ostiomeatal complex (▶ Fig. 3.14).

Care must be taken to respect the integrity of Schneider's membrane: rotating instruments allow more rapid completion of the osteotomy, but may carry a higher risk of membrane perforation. Conversely, piezoelectric instruments, although slower in removing bone along the osteotomy lines, are nontraumatic for soft tissues and may reduce the risk of membrane tears.[36] Once the outlining of the bony window is complete, the membrane is lifted with appropriately shaped blunt and sharp instruments, which are constantly kept in direct contact with the bone walls. Great care must be taken to maintain the integrity of the membrane, to avoid displacement of the grafting materials into the sinus, which represents one of the main causes of failure (▶ Fig. 3.15). See Section 3.4.3, Perforation of the Sinus Membrane, for further details. The membrane usually adheres most tenaciously to the maxillary sinus bone at the level of the anteroinferior border of the bony window. Consequently, great care must be taken during the elevation of this area.

Once the dissection is complete, the grafting material is inserted to fill the subsinusal space that has been created. The grafting material should be compacted but not excessively compressed into the cavity, as this maneuver may reduce the blood supply to the graft and consequently delay or inhibit the healing process, or it may lead to tearing of the sinus membrane.

Implants can be inserted at the same time as the sinus floor elevation procedure (generally speaking, when primary stability of the implant is guaranteed by the residual alveolar bone) or in a second stage, once the grafting material has been adequately integrated (generally 6–12 months later).

A resorbable membrane can be placed over the bony window to avoid dispersion of the grafting material and to improve the integration of the material.[29,37,38] The procedure is completed with a tension-free suture of the surgical flaps after periosteal releasing incisions.

3.4.2 Elevation of the Sinus Membrane through a Crestal Approach

The sinus lift procedure through a crestal approach is a site-specific surgical technique that allows vertical augmentation of the bone in the maxillary premolar and molar regions directly through the residual alveolar crest. Many authors have introduced small variations to this technique; however, the general principles described by the surgeons who first proposed it, Tatum[39] and Summers,[22] are still followed.

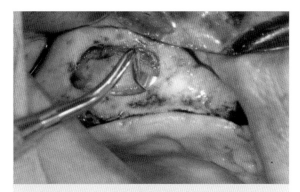

Fig. 3.15 Sinus lift via a lateral approach. Surgical access, antrostomy, and elevation of the sinus membrane with manual instruments.

The bone height of the residual alveolar ridge is measured on preoperative radiographs: a midcrestal incision and the exposure of only the alveolar crest is generally sufficient to gain enough access. The alveolar ridge cortex is perforated with a rotating instrument (e.g., a cylindrical bur with a 2-mm diameter) and osteotomes of progressively increasing diameter with a concave tip are then inserted and gently struck with a surgical mallet; this allows the collection of bone particles along the margins of the site and their compression at the apex. The tip of the final osteotome must fracture the floor of the maxillary sinus without perforating the sinus membrane, and the collected bone, pushed underneath the membrane, will induce its elevation. When the floor of the sinus has a particularly resistant cortex, it is advisable not to increase the power of the strikes as this could lead to perforation of the membrane (compromising the success of the procedure) and increase the postoperative discomfort (including complications such as vertigo). In such patients, it is preferable to erode the bony plate with a rotating bur or a piezoelectric instrument. As the autologous bone particles will be removed by these instruments, a biomaterial can be gently pushed upward through the implant site with an osteotome to obtain the planned vertical increase.[40,41] Finally, if the residual bone height of the crest guarantees primary stability of implants (generally, at least 4 mm), it is possible to insert them during the same session (▶ Fig. 3.16). The surgical procedure is completed by a flap suture.

Compared with the lateral approach, the crestal approach is theoretically less invasive: there is no need for elevation of wide flaps and no need to create a bony window in the lateral aspect of the maxillary sinus wall. However, it allows a lower increase in bone height and is a relatively blind technique. The surgeon, following a strict protocol and using specific instruments, has tactile control of the elevation of the sinus membrane, but no direct vision.

3.4.3 Complications

Accurate preoperative planning, including a meticulous medical and dental history and thorough radiological evaluation of the sinus anatomy, and surgical procedures

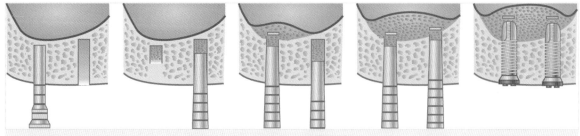

Fig. 3.16 Sinus lift through a crestal approach. Initial site preparation, preservation of the sinus floor, placement of the grafting material, fracture of the sinus floor with the final osteotome, and implant placement.

with well-defined protocols can significantly reduce the incidence of complications. However, as with any surgical procedure, maxillary sinus elevation does have potential complications, both intraoperative and postoperative, which can be summarized as follows:

• Perforation of the sinus membrane.
• Bleeding.
• Damage to adjacent tooth roots and risk to their vascular supply.
• Stasis of mucus in an inadequately lifted sinus.
• Pain and/or infraorbital nerve paresthesia.
• Wound dehiscence.
• Infection of the surgical site, sinusitis, and spread of infection to perisinusal spaces.
• Implant displacement or migration into the maxillary sinus.
• Vertigo.

Perforation of the Sinus Membrane

The preservation of sinus membrane integrity is key to success, as it provides stability and a good blood supply to the grafting material and prevents its dispersion into the maxillary sinus (▶ Fig. 3.17).

The risk of membrane perforation during preparation of the bony window, elevation of the membrane, positioning of the grafting material, and implant placement (if performed at the same stage), varies between 7% and 44%, with an average of approximately 10%.[24,42,43] This wide range is related to the surgeon's skill and experience, but also to anatomical features of the sinus cavity (e.g., sharp angles of the inferomesial wall of the sinus and the presence of septa) and the membrane thickness (▶ Fig. 3.18).

A retrospective study by von Arx et al[44] investigated the influence of factors that may increase the risk of membrane perforation during sinus lift using a lateral approach. Results showed that smoking, the presence of Underwood's septa, a residual alveolar ridge height of less than 4 mm, multiple edentulous segments, and a thin sinus membrane may increase this risk. As perforations may also occur in experienced hands during the outlining of osteotomies (in a lateral approach) or during its elevation, it is of the utmost importance to be able to deal with them.

Tearing of the membrane per se is not a problem if nothing is grafted into the subsinusal cavity created by sinus floor elevation, as the membrane can undergo spontaneous healing within a few weeks. However, problems may arise when grafting material is placed in the cavity: the presence of a perforation may allow the displacement of grafting material during surgery or its migration during a second stage.

Different scenarios may follow dispersion of the graft material into the sinus. The migrating graft particles may be incorporated into the mucous film and transported toward the ostium by mucociliary clearance. If the dimensions of the ostium (usually 7–11 mm in height and 2–6 mm in length) are adequate and the drainage mechanism provided by the ciliated epithelium is efficient, the particles can be expelled into the nasal cavity and then through the nasopharynx into the aerodigestive tract. Otherwise, secondary occlusion of the ostium and/or a lack of spontaneous drainage may lead to a reduction in sinus ventilation (with consequent lowering of the oxygen concentration and an increase in CO_2 concentration in the sinus), suspension of ciliary activity, stasis of the mucus, and a hyperplastic inflammatory reaction in the sinus membrane. All these factors will create an ideal environment for the growth of anaerobic bacteria and

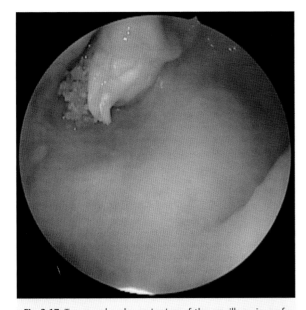

Fig. 3.17 Transnasal endoscopic view of the maxillary sinus of an anatomical specimen. The sinus membrane has been torn during a simulated maxillary sinus augmentation and repaired with a collagen membrane. Even though the repair is successful, simulating an excessive pressure during the graft-positioning maneuver causes the bony particulate to breach into the sinus.

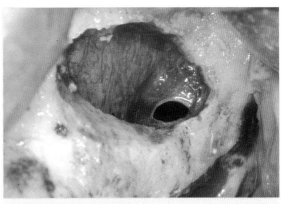

Fig. 3.18 Perforation of the sinus membrane.

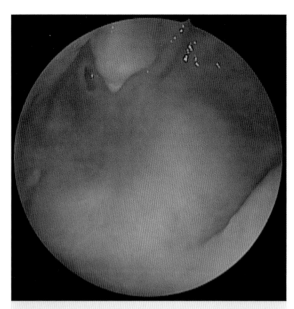

Fig. 3.19 Endonasal endoscopic view of the maxillary sinus of an anatomical specimen. A simulated sinus membrane tear repaired with a collagen membrane.

sinus infection. For these reasons, perforations should always be identified during surgery and immediately repaired (▶ Fig. 3.19).

In 2003, Fugazzotto and Vlassis[45] and Proussaefs and Lozada[46] classified sinus membrane perforations and proposed a protocol for their management. If the perforation is localized in the cranial portion of the bony window, it is advisable to reduce the tension of the membrane with blunt dissection in the lateral and caudal regions of the floor of the sinus: this maneuver will favor membrane sagging and spontaneous closure of the tear. If the perforation is localized laterally, increasing the dimensions of the bony window is indicated, to expose 4 to 5 mm of intact membrane and continue the dissection to let the mucosa sag into itself. When it is not possible to enlarge the margins of the bony window or when the tear is too large, performing a "pouch" technique is recommended. This involves positioning a resorbable collagen membrane over the perforation and on the bony sinus walls, creating a new cavity to contain the grafting material before it is placed. Mixing the graft with venous blood or autologous blood products such as platelet-rich plasma (PRP) may increase the stability and maneuverability of the graft and will reduce the risk of leakage of the material into the sinus through the perforated membrane.

Bleeding

As previously explained, one of the key requirements for a successful sinus lift is to preserve the integrity of Schneider's membrane. Working in a bloodless surgical field improves the view and facilitates surgical maneuvers. It is therefore crucial to choose a suitable flap, maintain its integrity, and perform a subperiosteal dissection, which will significantly reduce local bleeding.

Another source of bleeding that may interfere with the sinus grafting procedure when using a lateral approach is the alveolar antral artery, an anastomotic branch connecting the posterior superior alveolar artery and the infraorbital artery, described in Chapter 2 (p.16). This vessel, which delivers the blood supply to the antral mucosa and the thin anterolateral wall of the maxillary sinus, runs in the majority of patients in a horizontal direction in a canal located in the vestibular wall of the maxillary sinus, 6 to 20 mm cranial to the residual bone crest. In a minority of patients, the artery runs along the inner aspect of the wall. The vessel varies from 0.2 up to 3 mm in diameter and the canal is clearly visible on CT scans in approximately 80% of patients.[47,48]

Vessels with a very small (< 0.5 mm) diameter hardly interfere with the surgical procedure, but with vessels of larger diameter the bleeding can be significant and may lead to: (1) greater difficulty controlling the surgical field, in particular during the elevation of Schneider's membrane; (2) postoperative bleeding in the oral and/or nasal cavity; (3) postoperative bleeding with "wash-out" of the grafting material, which is dispersed outside the grafted area; (4) postoperative hematomas, which may lead to wound dehiscence and create an ideal environment for infection.

The design of the bony window must take into consideration the position of the artery and, if possible, the superior border of the window should be below the artery. If the artery cannot be avoided, it is important to preserve its integrity by using piezoelectric instruments or be ready to deal with a possible hemorrhage, which is generally easily controlled with compression, hemostatic agents, or diathermy. Only in the (albeit extremely rare) circumstances where larger vessels run along the inner aspect of the sinus wall, rather than in the bony canal on the lateral wall of the sinus as is normally the case, might ligation of the vessel be necessary.

Damage to Adjacent Tooth Roots and Risk to Their Vascular Supply

Expansion of the sinus can lead to a significant reduction of bone volume around the teeth in the posterior maxilla. Therefore, if preoperative CT scans do not show any alveolar bone surrounding the apices of the residual teeth, nerves and vessels supplying the dental pulp may run within Schneider's membrane. In this case, lifting the membrane may compromise the vascular and neural supply, causing necrosis of the dental pulp. It is advisable to always maintain a distance of 3 to 5 mm from the apices during dissection of the membrane, even if this inevitably leads to a reduction in the dimensions of bone augmentation.

Stasis of Mucus in the Inadequately Lifted Sinus

When performing a sinus lift, it is important to elevate the membrane up to the lateral nasal wall to allow the grafting material to acquire the correct conformation and receive a greater vascular supply from the bone walls. Incomplete dissection of the membrane can modify the anatomy of the sinus, producing areas with poor drainage of mucus toward the ostium and therefore increasing the risk of infection.[49]

Paresthesia of the Infraorbital Nerve

An incorrect flap design with vertical releasing incisions in the canine region, deep in the sulcus, or excessive traction with surgical retractors may induce a temporary or permanent paresthesia of the area innervated by the infraorbital nerve.

Wound Dehiscence

This usually occurs one or more weeks after surgery. The most important factor in minimizing this risk is a tension-free and water-tight suture, after adequate releasing incisions in the flap periosteum, particularly when the sinus grafting is associated with reconstruction of severely resorbed alveolar crests with only grafts or guided bone regeneration procedures. Other contributing factors are wearing fixed or mobile prostheses on the operated area within at least the first 6 to 8 weeks postoperatively and not following a soft diet for at least 2 weeks after surgery.

Dehiscence may be followed by superficial contamination of the underlying bone, caused by the intraoral microbial flora; however, antibiotic therapy and topical control with chlorhexidine mouthwashes or gels may be followed by spontaneous healing by secondary intention.

A second scenario is infection of the surgical site, which may also be followed by spread of the infection toward the maxillary and other paranasal sinuses, or even toward the cranial fossae. As the clinical implications are important, the next section of this textbook will be dedicated to this topic.

Infection of the Surgical Site, Sinusitis, and Spread of Infection to Perisinusal Spaces

Chronic or acute sinusitis is caused by colonization of the grafting material by pathogenic microorganisms. The contamination may occur during the sinus grafting procedure (from the patient's saliva, nonsterile grafting material, or surgical instruments) or in the postoperative period, following the dehiscence of the surgical wound or tears in Schneider's membrane. The latter may lead to migration of the grafting material into the sinus (followed by a foreign body reaction and infection) or contamination of the graft by nasal bacteria without evident displacement of the graft into the sinus.

As highlighted by Testori et al,[50] it is fundamentally important to determine whether the bacterial contamination of the grafting material, and the resulting infection, remains limited to the surgical site (between the floor of the sinus and Schneider's membrane) or if it involves the entire antral cavity. The differential diagnosis can be performed with computed tomography. In the first scenario, the CT scan shows a hyperplasic inflammatory thickening of Schneider's membrane, but with normal patency of the ostiomeatal complex and normal ventilation of the sinus. In the second scenario, the scan shows a massive opacification of the antral cavity due to dispersion of the grafting material within the sinus, with loss of the physiological mechanisms of drainage and ventilation.

A correct diagnosis is crucial for adequate management of this complication. Therefore, 3 weeks after the procedure, if the normal postoperative symptoms following sinus lift (edema, bruising, mild pain or discomfort, minimal bleeding from the wound or the nose) persist or worsen, a radiological examination is recommended. Treatment modalities differ significantly, depending on the diagnosis, as described in the following scenarios.

Scenario 1

If a patient complains of the aforementioned symptoms with evidence of pus discharging from the surgical wound, the grafting material is autologous particulate bone, and the CT scan shows a normally ventilated sinus with no evidence of ostiomeatal complex abnormality and a well-delimited infection under Schneider's membrane, prescription of a medical treatment is recommended (▶ Table 3.2) together with close follow-up. The symptoms should resolve within 2 weeks. This conservative approach is possible with autologous material as early vascularization allows antibiotics to reach the surgical site and be effective in the infected area (▶ Fig. 3.20).

Table 3.2 Drug chart for sinus lift complications

Patients not allergic to penicillin	1 g amoxicillin/clavulanate orally 3 times per day plus metronidazole 500 mg orally 3 times per day
Patients allergic to penicillin	500 mg levofloxacin orally 2 times per day for up to 72 hours after remission of symptoms (this usually requires 7–10 days)

Scenario 2

Three weeks after a sinus lift, typical postoperative signs and symptoms persist. Gradually, other symptoms arise, such as increasing pain and mild nasal obstruction, while oral fistulae, oral wound dehiscence, and pus and grafting material discharging in the oral cavity may be apparent. The CT scan shows the presence of the graft (autologous or heterologous), well contained underneath Schneider's membrane, and the sinus still normally ventilated, despite a reactive thickening of the mucosa.

Management consists of antibiotic therapy (▶ Table 3.2) combined with partial or complete surgical removal of the infected graft via an intraoral approach. Complete resolution of the symptoms generally occurs within 2 weeks.

Scenario 3

The signs and symptoms described above are associated with leakage of the grafting material into the sinus. The physiological mechanisms of clearance and ventilation of the sinus are compromised and an acute sinusitis develops with edema, swelling, pain, pus discharge from the nose and/or the surgical wound, dehiscence of the wound, and discharge of grafting material in the oral cavity (▶ Fig. 3.21a).

A multidisciplinary approach with systemic medical therapy (▶ Table 3.2) and complete surgical removal of the grafting material via a combined intraoral and transnasal functional endoscopic sinus surgery (FESS) approach is recommended[25,50] (▶ Fig. 3.21b) (group I, class 1a).

In order to prevent these complications, it is advisable to perform this procedure following strict protocols, using sterile instruments and adequate materials to avoid intraoperative contamination. Prescription of a perioperative antibiotic therapy is also recommended (▶ Table 3.3).[50–52]

It is worth noting that sinus infection, if not adequately treated, may lead to major complications, including osteomyelitis, orbital cellulitis, and septic venous thrombosis with the risk of loss of vision.

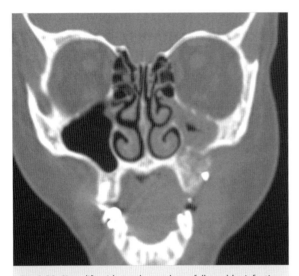

Fig. 3.20 Sinus lift with autologous bone followed by infection of the graft. A CT scan performed 30 days postsurgery shows significant mucosal edema with residual air pockets. A broad-spectrum antibiotic regimen resolved the infection and implants were placed 4 months later.

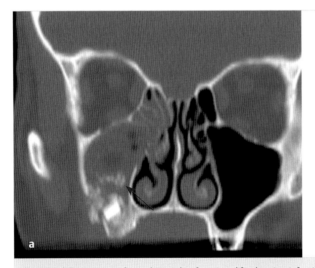
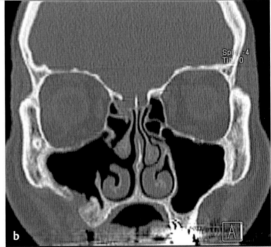

Fig. 3.21 (a) CT scan performed 3 weeks after sinus lift, showing infection of the grafting material (*arrow*) not contained by Schneider's membrane, with right ethmoidal and maxillary sinusitis. (b) CT scan performed 6 months later, showing resolution of signs of sinusitis following a multidisciplinary approach to treatment, consisting of removal of the infected graft via an intraoral approach and functional endoscopic sinus surgery (FESS).

Implant Displacement or Migration into the Maxillary Sinus

In 2008, Pjetursson et al[29] published a systematic review of sinus grafting procedures and survival rates of implants placed in the grafted areas. Forty-eight papers were included, reporting on 12,020 implants placed in more than 4,000 patients treated with a sinus grafting procedure. An overall survival rate of implants of 90.1% after a 3-year follow-up was recorded. Similar results have been reported by other systematic reviews on the same topic.[24,30] In conclusion, the literature demonstrates that endosseous implants placed in association with sinus grafting present high survival rates, consistent with those reported for implants placed in native bone.

Implants can be placed either at the same stage as the sinus grafting procedure, or in a second stage, once the grafted material is adequately integrated and consolidated (6–12 months after the grafting procedure, on average).

Table 3.3 Perioperative drug therapy in sinus lift patients to prevent complications

Patients not allergic to penicillin	
Prophylaxis	1 g amoxicillin/clavulanate orally 2 times per day, starting 24 h prior to surgery
Postoperative therapy	1 g amoxicillin/clavulanate orally 3 times per day for 7 days
Patients allergic to penicillin	
Prophylaxis	250 mg clarithromycin orally 2 times per day plus 500 mg metronidazole orally 3 times per day, starting 24 h prior to surgery
Postoperative therapy	250 mg clarithromycin orally 2 times per day plus 500 mg metronidazole orally for 7 days

When the anatomical conditions are favorable (i.e., there is enough residual bone in the alveolar crest to guarantee primary stability of implants), the surgeon may decide to insert implants at the same time as the sinus grafting procedure. Briefly, once the sinus membrane has been lifted, the implant sites are prepared according to the standard procedures for implant placement in native bone (generally speaking, a sequence of burs of increasing diameter). It is advisable to protect the membrane with periosteal elevators during this phase. The grafting material is then positioned in contact with the lateral nasal wall and in the anterior and posterior sinus recesses, and subsequently the implants are positioned. Finally, the residual gaps are filled with the grafting material up to the vestibular sinus wall. This sequence allows constant visual control of the different steps and avoids overfilling of the surgical site, which could otherwise lead to sinus membrane perforation.

When the expansion of the sinus is such that the residual alveolar bone height is limited (<3 mm) and/or the quality of the bone is poor, the lack of primary stability of the implants and unidentified perforations of the sinus membrane can induce leakage of the graft and the implants into the maxillary sinus, potentially causing sinusitis and obstruction of the ostiomeatal complex. Implants that have migrated into the sinus (as well as any grafting material) (▸ Fig. 3.22) must immediately be removed via an intraoral and/or endoscopic transnasal approach.

Vertigo

Postoperative benign paroxysmal positional vertigo (BPPV) may be a complication following a sinus lift procedure via a crestal approach, caused by the percussion of the osteotomes with the mallet; this may occur in approximately 3% of the patients.[30,53]

The symptoms are specific and consist of recurrent vertigo lasting a few seconds and associated with a change in head position. The pathophysiology of the disease is based on the release of otoliths from macules and the

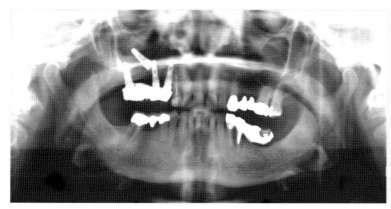

Fig. 3.22 Panoramic radiograph showing grafting material and an implant displaced into the sinus.

subsequent displacement of these otoliths in a semicircular canal. The symptoms usually disappear spontaneously within a few days or with the help of an otorhinolaryngologist who can perform a liberation maneuver.[54]

References

[1] Patel NA, Ferguson BJ. Odontogenic sinusitis: an ancient but underappreciated cause of maxillary sinusitis. Curr Opin Otolaryngol Head Neck Surg 2012; 20: 24–28

[2] Van Dyke TE, Vaikuntam J. Neutrophil function and dysfunction in periodontal disease. In: Williams RC, Yukna RA, Newman MG, eds. Current Opinion in Periodontology. Philadelphia: Current Science; 1994:19–27

[3] Ryan GB, Majno G. Acute inflammation. A review. Am J Pathol 1977; 86: 183–276

[4] Baumgartner JC, Falkler WA Jr. Bacteria in the apical 5 mm of infected root canals. J Endod 1991; 17: 380–383

[5] Sundqvist G. Bacteriological Studies of Necrotic Dental Pulps [PhD thesis]. Umeaˆ, Sweden: University of Umeaˆ; 1976

[6] Fabricius L, Dahlén G, Ohman AE, Möller AJR. Predominant indigenous oral bacteria isolated from infected root canals after varied times of closure. Scand J Dent Res 1982; 90: 134–144

[7] Loesche WJ, Gusberti F, Mettraux G, Higgins T, Syed S. Relationship between oxygen tension and subgingival bacterial flora in untreated human periodontal pockets. Infect Immun 1983; 42: 659–667

[8] Carlsson J. Microbiology of plaque-associated periodontal disease. In: Lindhe J, ed. Textbook of Clinical Periodontology. 2nd ed. Copenhagen: Munksgaard; 1989

[9] Lev M, Keudell KC, Milford AF. Succinate as a growth factor for Bacteroides melaninogenicus. J Bacteriol 1971; 108: 175–178

[10] Toller P. Origin and growth of cysts of the jaws. Ann R Coll Surg Engl 1967; 40: 306–336

[11] Harris M. Odontogenic cyst growth and prostaglandin-induced bone resorption. Ann R Coll Surg Engl 1978; 60: 85–91

[12] Cohen S, Burns RC. Pathways of the Pulp. 8th ed. St Louis, MO: Mosby Elsevier; 2002

[13] Quiney RE, Brimble E, Hodge M. Maxillary sinusitis from dental osseointegrated implants. J Laryngol Otol 1990; 104: 333–334

[14] Alkan A, Celebi N, Baş B. Acute maxillary sinusitis associated with internal sinus lifting: report of a case. Eur J Dent 2008; 2: 69–72

[15] Li J, Wang HL. Common implant-related advanced bone grafting complications: classification, etiology, and management. Implant Dent 2008; 17: 389–401

[16] Brånemark PI. Osseointegration and its experimental background. J Prosthet Dent 1983; 50: 399–410

[17] Schroeder A, van der Zypen E, Stich H, Sutter F. The reactions of bone, connective tissue, and epithelium to endosteal implants with titanium-sprayed surfaces. J Maxillofac Surg 1981; 9: 15–25

[18] Esposito M, Murray-Curtis L, Grusovin MG, Coulthard P, Worthington HV. Interventions for replacing missing teeth: different types of dental implants. Cochrane Database Syst Rev 2007; 17: CD003815

[19] Lambert FE, Weber HP, Susarla SM, Belser UC, Gallucci GO. Descriptive analysis of implant and prosthodontic survival rates with fixed implant-supported rehabilitations in the edentulous maxilla. J Periodontol 2009; 80: 1220–1230

[20] Cawood JI, Howell RA. A classification of the edentulous jaws. Int J Oral Maxillofac Surg 1988; 17: 232–236

[21] Boyne PJ, James RA. Grafting of the maxillary sinus floor with autogenous marrow and bone. J Oral Surg 1980; 38: 613–616

[22] Summers RB. A new concept in maxillary implant surgery: the osteotome technique. Compendium 1994; 15: 152, 154–156, 158 passim, quiz 162

[23] Chiapasco M, Zaniboni M, Rimondini L. Dental implants placed in grafted maxillary sinuses: a retrospective analysis of clinical outcome according to the initial clinical situation and a proposal of defect classification. Clin Oral Implants Res 2008; 19: 416–428

[24] Chiapasco M, Casentini P, Zaniboni M. Bone augmentation procedures in implant dentistry. Int J Oral Maxillofac Implants 2009; 24 Suppl: 237–259

[25] Chiapasco M, Felisati G, Maccari A, Borloni R, Gatti F, Di Leo F. The management of complications following displacement of oral implants in the paranasal sinuses: a multicenter clinical report and proposed treatment protocols. Int J Oral Maxillofac Surg 2009; 38 Suppl: 1273–1278

[26] Brånemark PI, Adell R, Albrektsson T, Lekholm U, Lindström J, Rockler B. An experimental and clinical study of osseointegrated implants penetrating the nasal cavity and maxillary sinus. J Oral Maxillofac Surg 1984; 42: 497–505

[27] Regev E, Smith RA, Perrott DH, Pogrel MA. Maxillary sinus complications related to endosseous implants. Int J Oral Maxillofac Implants 1995; 10: 451–461

[28] Tatum OH. Maxillary sinus grafting for endosseous implants. Lecture presented at: Annual Meeting of the Alabama Implant Study Group; April 1977; Birmingham, AL

[29] Pjetursson BE, Tan WC, Zwahlen M, Lang NP. A systematic review of the success of sinus floor elevation and survival of implants inserted in combination with sinus floor elevation. J Clin Periodontol 2008; 35 Suppl: 216–240

[30] Del Fabbro M, Wallace SS, Testori T. Long-term implant survival in the grafted maxillary sinus: a systematic review. Int J Periodontics Restorative Dent 2013; 33: 773–783

[31] Jensen OT, Shulman LB, Block MS, Iacono VJ. Report of the sinus consensus conference of 1996. Int J Oral Maxillofac Implants 1998; 13 Suppl: 11–45

[32] Urist MR. Bone: formation by autoinduction. Science 1965; 150: 893–899

[33] Jensen OT, Sennerby L. Histologic analysis of clinically retrieved titanium microimplants placed in conjunction with maxillary sinus floor augmentation. Int J Oral Maxillofac Implants 1998; 13: 513–521

[34] Cordioli G, Majzoub ZI. Biovetri in chirurgia orale. In: Testori T, Weinstein R, Del Fabbro M. La chirurgia del seno mascellare e le alternative terapeutiche. Viterbo, Italy: ACME; 2005:196–207

[35] Avila-Ortiz G, Wang HL, Galindo-Moreno P, Misch CE, Rudek I, Neiva R. Influence of lateral window dimensions on vital bone formation following maxillary sinus augmentation. Int J Oral Maxillofac Implants 2012; 27: 1230–1238

[36] Vercellotti T, De Paoli S, Nevins M. The piezoelectric bony window osteotomy and sinus membrane elevation: introduction of a new technique for simplification of the sinus augmentation procedure. Int J Periodontics Restorative Dent 2001; 21: 561–567

[37] Tarnow DP, Wallace SS, Froum SJ, Rohrer MD, Cho SC. Histologic and clinical comparison of bilateral sinus floor elevations with and with-

out barrier membrane placement in 12 patients: Part 3 of an ongoing prospective study. Int J Periodontics Restorative Dent 2000; 20: 117–125

[38] Tawil G, Mawla M. Sinus floor elevation using a bovine bone mineral (Bio-Oss) with or without the concomitant use of a bilayered collagen barrier (Bio-Gide): a clinical report of immediate and delayed implant placement. Int J Oral Maxillofac Implants 2001; 16: 713–721

[39] Tatum H Jr. Maxillary and sinus implant reconstructions. Dent Clin North Am 1986; 30: 207–229

[40] Nkenke E, Kloss F, Wiltfang J et al. Histomorphometric and fluorescence microscopic analysis of bone remodelling after installation of implants using an osteotome technique. Clin Oral Implants Res 2002; 13: 595–602

[41] Nkenke E, Schlegel A, Schultze-Mosgau S, Neukam FW, Wiltfang J. The endoscopically controlled osteotome sinus floor elevation: a preliminary prospective study. Int J Oral Maxillofac Implants 2002; 17: 557–566

[42] Schwartz-Arad D, Herzberg R, Dolev E. The prevalence of surgical complications of the sinus graft procedure and their impact on implant survival. J Periodontol 2004; 75: 511–516

[43] Jensen OT, Shulman LB, Block MS, Iacono VJ. Report of the sinus consensus conference of 1996. Int J Oral Maxillofac Implants 1998; 13 Suppl: 11–45

[44] von Arx T, Fodich I, Bornstein MM, Jensen SS. Perforation of the sinus membrane during sinus floor elevation: a retrospective study of frequency and possible risk factors. Int J Oral Maxillofac Implants 2014; 29: 718–726

[45] Fugazzotto PA, Vlassis J. A simplified classification and repair system for sinus membrane perforations. J Periodontol 2003; 74: 1534–1541

[46] Proussaefs P, Lozada J. The "Loma Linda pouch": a technique for repairing the perforated sinus membrane. Int J Periodontics Restorative Dent 2003; 23: 593–597

[47] Rosano G, Taschieri S, Gaudy JF, Weinstein T, Del Fabbro M. Maxillary sinus vascular anatomy and its relation to sinus lift surgery. Clin Oral Implants Res 2011; 22: 711–715

[48] Apostolakis D, Bissoon AK. Radiographic evaluation of the superior alveolar canal: measurements of its diameter and of its position in relation to the maxillary sinus floor: a cone beam computerized tomography study. Clin Oral Implants Res 2014; 25: 553–559

[49] Levi PA, Marcuschamer E. Avoiding and managing complications for the lateral window technique. In: Kao DWK, ed. Clinical Maxillary Sinus Elevation Surgery. Ames, IA: John Wiley & Sons; 2014:79–104

[50] Testori T, Drago L, Wallace SS et al. Prevention and treatment of postoperative infections after sinus elevation surgery: clinical consensus and recommendations. Int J Dent 2012; 2012: 365809

[51] Esposito M, Cannizzaro G, Bozzoli P et al. Effectiveness of prophylactic antibiotics at placement of dental implants: a pragmatic multicentre placebo-controlled randomised clinical trial. Eur J Oral Implantology 2010; 3: 135–143

[52] Esposito M, Grusovin MG, Loli V, Coulthard P, Worthington HV. Does antibiotic prophylaxis at implant placement decrease early implant failures? A Cochrane systematic review. Eur J Oral Implantology 2010; 3: 101–110

[53] Peñarrocha M, Pérez H, Garciá A, Guarinos J. Benign paroxysmal positional vertigo as a complication of osteotome expansion of the maxillary alveolar ridge. J Oral Maxillofac Surg 2001; 59: 106–107

[54] Sammartino G, Mariniello M, Scaravilli MS. Benign paroxysmal positional vertigo following closed sinus floor elevation procedure: mallet osteotomes vs. screwable osteotomes. A triple blind randomized controlled trial. Clin Oral Implants Res 2011; 22: 669–672

Chapter 4

Microbiology of Odontogenic Sinusitis

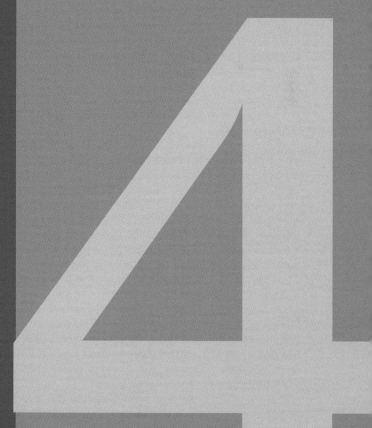

4 Microbiology of Odontogenic Sinusitis

Lorenzo Drago and Alberto Maria Saibene

Contents Overview

The aim of this chapter is to provide a quick microbiological and infectivological reference for sinonasal conditions resulting from dental causes. The first part of the chapter is a state of the art review on the current knowledge of the oral microbiome, which is of prime importance in dealing with SCDDT: microbial composition, technical analytical approaches, oral and non-oral related diseases, and also future developments are taken into account.

The second part of the chapter will focus on sinonasal complications of dental disease and treatment by analyzing in detail their two main clinical manifestations: bacterial sinusitis and fungal sinusitis. Both pathogens of interest and physiopathogenetic mechanics are depicted.

4.1 Introduction: Oral Microbiome and SCDDT

Chronic rhinosinusitis (CRS) is a well-defined nosological entity: most of its pathogenetic features have been described in detail and its microbiology has been addressed more than adequately in a number of works. These are summarized in the EPOS, the biennial position paper on rhinosinusitis by the European Rhinologic Society; the most recent edition was published in 2012.[1]

In contrast, odontogenic sinusitis is an ill-defined condition and reliable information concerning its microbiological features is scarce to nonexistent, with abundant small studies often lacking in patient numbers or methodological strength.

Nevertheless, there is one major point on which nearly all authors who have studied odontogenic sinusitis and sinonasal complications of dental disease or treatment (SCDDT) agree: odontogenic sinusitis and CRS represent two distinct disorders, which share many signs and symptoms but begin and develop in markedly different ways. One of the most important features of odontogenic infections is—as the name implies—the major role that the oral microbiome plays in the sinuses. Dental conditions and dental procedures act as a "Trojan horse," allowing a massive transfer of pathogens into the sinonasal cavities, often modifying the sinonasal physiology. These oral pathogens are unable to cause sinonasal infections under normal conditions, but when present in high numbers in the less well-defended sinonasal cavity they cause distinctive infections, both bacterial and fungal, with viruses retaining only a marginal role.

This chapter will therefore focus firstly on the oral microbiome, while the unique microbiology of odontogenic sinusitis is analyzed in the second part.

4.2 Human Oral Microbiota

4.2.1 Definition

The microorganisms found in the human oral cavity have been referred to as the oral microflora, oral microbiota, or oral microbiome. The oral cavity includes several distinct microbial habitats, including the teeth, gingival sulcus, attached gingiva, tongue, cheeks, lips, and hard and soft palate. Contiguous with the oral cavity are the tonsils, pharynx, esophagus, eustachian tube, middle ear, trachea, lungs, nasal passages, and sinuses. The human oral microbiota can be defined as all the microorganisms that are found on or in the human oral cavity and its contiguous extensions, stopping at the distal esophagus.[2]

4.2.2 Microbial Composition

The oral ecosystem is home to various human symbionts, including viruses, protozoa, fungi, archaea, and bacteria.[3]

A range of viruses can be found in the mouth; these are primarily disease-associated. Herpes viruses, hepatitis viruses, HPV, HIV, HTLV-I, and many others have been detected in salivary samples of affected individuals.[4] A survey of the oral virome in five healthy subjects revealed that the majority of virus sequences detected had homology with bacteriophages.[5]

Two protozoon species are found as part of the normal oral microbiota, *Entamoeba gingivalis* and *Trichomonas tenax*, which are regarded as harmless saprophytes.

A study of the oral mycobiota found 85 fungal genera in the mouths of 20 healthy individuals. The predominant genera were *Candida, Cladosporium, Aureobasidium, Saccharomycetales, Aspergillus, Fusarium*, and *Cryptococcus*.[6]

Among the prokaryote species that are present in the human oral cavity, 49% are officially named, 17% unnamed (but cultivated), and 34% are known only as uncultivated phylotypes. Representatives of the Archaea are restricted to a few taxa in the genus *Methanobrevibacter*, while around 1,000 bacterial species from at least 10 phyla have been found (▶ Table 4.1). The bacterial community found in the oral cavity is highly complex and is considered to be the second most complex in the body, after the colon.[7] Within the mouth, different surfaces have been shown to be colonized by distinct bacterial communities.[8]

Individuals' oral microbiomes are highly specific at the species level,[9] while there are similarities at the genus level.[10] The human oral microbiome shows few geographical differences,[11] suggesting that diet and environment do not significantly influence the composition of the oral microbiota and that the host is the primary determinant.

Table 4.1 Human oral microbiota taxonomic hierarchy

Domain	Phylum	Class
Archea	Euryarchaeota	Methanobacteria
Bacteria	Actinobacteria	Actinobacteria
	Bacteroidetes	Bacteroidia, Bacteroidetes, Flavobacteria
	Chlamydiae	Chlamydiae
	Chloroflexi	Chloroflexia
	Firmicutes	Bacilli, Clostridia, Erysipelotrichia
	Fusobacteria	Fusobacteria
	GN02	GN02
	Proteobacteria	Alphaproteobacteria, Betaproteobacteria, Deltaproteobacteria, Epsilonproteobacteria, Gammaproteobacteria
	Spirochaetes	Spirochaetia
	SR1	SR1
	Synergistetes	Synergistia
	Tenericutes	Mollicutes
	TM7	TM7

Note: Human oral microbiota taxonomic hierarchy is presented down to class level. Firmicutes, Bacteroidetes, Proteobacteria, Actinobacteria, Spirochaetes, and Fusobacteria account for approximately 96% of species. GN02, SR1, and TM7 represent uncultured divisions.

4.2.3 Technical Approaches

For decades, assessment of the microbiota of the human body was limited to species that could be isolated from laboratory cultures. Oral bacteria are particularly difficult to identify by conventional means because the majority are obligate anaerobes, slow-growing and unreactive in biochemical tests. The use of culture-independent methods for determining the composition of the microbiota, particularly molecular methods based on the comparison of small subunit (16S) ribosomal RNA genes, is providing a deeper analysis. The adoption of such methods has confirmed that there are a large number of uncultured bacterial species among the oral microbiota. These include representatives of the phyla Bacteroidetes, Firmicutes, Spirochaetes, and Sysergistetes, as well as entire divisions, such as GN02, SR1, and TM7, with no confirmed cultivable representatives.

New possibilities were opened up during the last decade with the advent of high-throughput genome sequencing, also known as next-generation sequencing (NGS). The major advantages of NGS are the high throughput, the relatively low cost, and the availability of sequencing facilities.[12] The interpretation of NGS data is the major

challenge as it can be undermined at numerous stages, including sample collection and storage, DNA extraction, choice of algorithms for data processing and statistical analysis, and by PCR bias and sequencing errors.

One of the most recent high-throughput sequencing platforms, the Ion-Torrent PGM[13] (Life Technologies, Carlsbad, California, USA), is just starting to be used in studies assessing human-associated microbiomes, including two for oral microbiota.[14,15] One study evaluated the temporal shifts in bacterial communities between periodontitis patients treated by scaling and root planing (SRP) alone versus SRP with adjunctive antibiotics,[15] while the other assessed the impact on the overall structure of the salivary microbiota of a short-term probiotic intervention.[14]

Species-level identification may not be sufficient, however, because of the genetic heterogeneity within species and the environmental influence on phenotype. The next step will be a combination of phylogenetic, metagenomic, transcriptomic, proteomic, and metabolomic approaches.

4.2.4 Oral Diseases

Oral microbes live primarily as complex polymicrobial communities, commonly called *biofilms* or, more specifically, *dental plaque*. Biofilms allow bacteria to live in a nutrient-rich milieu that is protected from environmental insults, antimicrobial agents, and frictional forces. In a state of good health, equilibrium exists between microorganisms and the host immune response. Under certain circumstances (e.g., a change in immune status) a shift occurs in the resident microflora, transforming this community from a commensal to a pathogenic one.

The microbiota of the mouth are responsible for two major oral diseases, dental caries and periodontal diseases, in addition to a number of other oral diseases including endodontic infections and alveolar osteitis. However, caries and periodontitis are not infectious diseases in the classical sense, because they result from a complex interaction between microbiota, host susceptibility, and environmental factors.

Dental caries is the dissolution of tooth structure caused by the organic acids produced during the fermentation of dietary carbohydrates by oral bacteria. A high level of acid production decreases the buffering capacity of saliva, leading to a reduction in pH and a shift in the composition of the oral microbiota to one enriched in aciduric species.[16] These species continue to produce acids under acidic conditions, thus exacerbating the damage to dental hard tissues. *Streptococcus mutans* and lactobacilli have been studied intensively for their cariogenic properties. Recently, members of the genera *Bifidobacterium*, *Propionibacterium*, and *Scardovia* have also been found to be associated with caries.[17,18]

Periodontitis appears to result from an inappropriate inflammatory reaction to the normal microbiota,

Table 4.2 Bacteria associated with periodontal diseases

Disease	Oral species detected
Gingivitis	*Actinomyces viscosus, Streptococcus* spp., *Parvimonas micra, Campylobacter gracilis, Fusobacterium nucleatum, Prevotella intermedia, Veillonella* spp.
Chronic periodontitis	*Porphyromonas gingivalis, Tannerella forsythia, Prevotella intermedia, Campylobacter rectus, Eikenella corrodens, Fusobacterium nucleatum, Aggregatibacter actinomycetemcomitans, Parvimonas micra, Treponema* spp.
Localized aggressive periodontitis	*Aggregatibacter actinomycetemcomitans, Porphyromonas gingivalis, Eikenella corrodens, Campylobacter rectus*
Generalized aggressive periodontitis	*Porphyromonas gingivalis, Tannerella forsythia, Prevotella intermedia, Campylobacter rectus, Eikenella corrodens, Fusobacterium nucleatum, Aggregatibacter actinomycetemcomitans, Parvimonas micra, Treponema* spp.
Necrotizing ulcerative gingivitis	*Treponema putidum, Rothia dentocariosa, Treponema* spp., *Achromobacter* spp., *Propionibacterium acnes, Capnocytophaga* spp., *Prevotella intermedia*
Periodontal abscess	*Fusobacterium nucleatum, Prevotella intermedia, Parvimonas micra, Tannerella forsythia, Campylobacter rectus, Porphyromonas gingivalis*

Source: Adapted from Kumar et al 2013.[19]

exacerbated by the presence of various disease-associated bacterial species. The host responds to pathogenic colonization with a florid immune response, leading to the breakdown of the attachment between the tooth and the supporting tissues, loss of alveolar bone, and deepening of the gingival sulcus, or "periodontal pocket." Different periodontal diseases have different profiles of associated bacteria. A list of the most common bacterial species detected is presented in ▶ Table 4.2.

4.2.5 Nonoral Diseases

The oral microbiota has long been known to be a reservoir for infection at other body sites. The periodontal pocket provides a protected environment, rich in blood-derived nutrients, and thus acts as a reservoir for pathogens. The proximity of bacteria to the vascular supply of the periodontium and the breakdown of epithelial integrity during the progression of periodontitis predisposes to states of bacteremia when the biofilm is disrupted. Oral bacteria and bacterial products can metastasize to nonoral sites during dental procedures. In most patients, this bacteremia is transient and the microorganisms are eliminated from the circulation. However, in certain patients, especially individuals with a compromised immune system, the oral microorganisms may colonize nonoral sites, leading to disease. Bacterial products (e.g., lipopolysaccharide and endotoxin) are also released into the systemic circulation and may trigger inflammatory responses in the target organs.

A growing body of evidence has implicated human oral microbiota in the etiology of various systemic diseases, including cardiovascular diseases, adverse pregnancy outcomes, respiratory tract infections, and many others (▶ Table 4.3). *Aggregatibacter actinomycetemcomitans* and *Porphyromonas gingivalis*, periodontopathic bacteria that are unique to the oral cavity and may disseminate to other body sites, are associated with the best documented forms of dental focal infection.

Conversely, recent studies have shown that the composition of the oral microbiota is sensitive to a number of systemic disease states of the host,[20–23] suggesting that oral microbiomic profiles could be used as noninvasive and readily accessible diagnostic biomarkers for other diseases.

4.2.6 Future Directions

The microbial etiology of diseases has evolved along with advances in technology. New, uncultivated, disease-associated microbial species have been recognized, together with risk factors that modulate host–bacterial interactions. Many of these discoveries hold promise for new prevention and treatment modalities.

In the case of the oral microbiota, which includes genera (e.g., *Porphyromonas, Aggregatibacter,* and *Tannerella*) comprising species strongly associated with diseases or health status, species-level identification is a significant issue. However, species-level identification may not be sufficient, because a wide heterogeneity is present within species. For instance, it seems that only select subtypes of a given species in the oral microbiota (e.g., *Fusobacterium nucleatum* subsp. *animalis* and subsp. *polymorphum* and *Streptococcus mutans* non-c serotypes) are prone to extraoral translocation resulting in disease. These findings highlight the importance of identifying potential pathogens at the subtype level for accurate prediction of disease potential.

The influence of environmental factors on phenotype introduces a further layer of complexity. The interaction

Table 4.3 Summary of oral species implicated in extraoral diseases

Disease	Oral species detected
Cardiovascular diseases	*Aggregatibacter actinomycetemcomitans, Campylobacter rectus, Chlamydia pneumoniae, Eikenella corrodens, Fusobacterium necrophorum, Fusobacterium nucleatum, Porphyromonas gingivalis, Prevotella intermedia, Streptococcus mitis, Streptococcus mutans, Streptococcus oralis, Tannerella forsythia, Treponema denticola*
Adverse pregnancy outcomes	*Bergeyella* spp., *Campylobacter rectus, Capnocytophaga* spp., *Eikenella corrodens, Fusobacterium nucleatum, Peptostreptococcus micros, Porphyromonas gingivalis, Prevotella intermedia, Prevotella nigrescens, Rothia dentocariosa, Streptococcus mutans, Tannerella forsythia, Treponema denticola*
Rheumatoid arthritis	*Fusobacterium nucleatum, Porphyromonas gingivalis, Prevotella intermedia, Prevotella melaninogenica, Serratia proteamaculans, Tannerella forsythia*
Inflammatory bowel disease and colorectal cancer	*Campylobacter concisus, Fusobacterium nucleatum, Streptococcus mutans*
Respiratory tract infections	*Staphylococcus aureus, Pseudomonas aeruginosa, Acinetobacter* spp., *Candida albicans*, enteric species
Meningitis or brain abscesses	*Campylobacter rectus, Fusobacterium necrophorum, Fusobacterium nucleatum, Porphyromonas gingivalis, Streptococcus intermedius*
Lung, liver, or splenic abscesses	*Fusobacterium necrophorum, Fusobacterium nucleatum, Porphyromonas gingivalis, Prevotella* spp., *Treponema denticola*
Appendicitis	*Fusobacterium necrophorum, Fusobacterium nucleatum*

Source: Adapted from Han and Wang 2013.[24]

between the human host and the microbiota is fundamental, but has rarely been studied. The first model of the human–microbial oral interactome, obtained using a computational prediction method, was published in 2014.[25]

In conclusion, functional rather than phylogenetic characterization, taking into account environmental influences, may be required in order to fully dissect oral host–microbiome interactions relevant to health and disease. The advent of NGS is providing vast amounts of new data, but caution is necessary as interpretation of this data is very challenging.

4.3 Pathogens

The microbiology of odontogenic sinusitis is extremely varied and strikingly different from other types of sinusitis, whether acute or chronic, for several reasons: (1) infections are most often polymicrobial, including pathogens of oral and sinonasal origin[26]; (2) an anaerobic flora is much more prevalent[27]; and (3) two biological kingdoms, bacteria and fungi, play an important role.[28] At present, clear information concerning the role of different pathogens in different groups and classes of SCDDT is not available: "odontogenic etiology" describes a single continuous, though extensive, microbiological scenario.

This section of this chapter will focus on the microbial flora of odontogenic sinusitis, discussing separately the features of bacterial and fungal infections.

4.3.1 Bacteria

An examination of scientific papers discussing the microbiology of acute and chronic maxillary sinusitis not associated with an odontogenic origin reveals that there is an almost universal consensus regarding the microbial flora: in the acute setting major pathogens are aerobic and facultative bacteria, most notably, *Streptococcus pneumoniae*, *Haemophilus influenzae*, and *Moraxella catarrhalis*.[29] In contrast, in chronic sinonasal conditions anaerobic bacteria predominate in 30–60% of patients.[30,31]

On the other hand, there is a lack of consensus concerning the microbiology of odontogenic sinusitis. Many studies include only a small number of patients, and so do not allow for a thorough assessment of the microbiology of this type of infection. Even the selection of patients for inclusion in each study introduces a disadvantage for studies of odontogenic sinusitis, because researchers still do not share a common overall definition of this condition.[32]

Itzhak Brook is one the most devoted researchers in the field of odontogenic sinusitis microbiology. In one of his most complete works, he shares his 30-year experience of studying the aerobic and anaerobic microbiology of acute and chronic maxillary sinusitis associated with odontogenic infection and demonstrates the peculiar aerobic and anaerobic microbiological features of such conditions.[33]

The microbial flora in odontogenic sinusitis appears radically different from acute rhinosinusitis (ARS) and

Table 4.4 Notable bacterial species in nonodontogenic and odontogenic sinusitis

Type of sinusitis	Aerobes	Anaerobes
Nonodontogenic sinusitis	*Staphylococcus aureus*, *S. epidermidis*, coagulase-negative *Staphylococcus* spp., *Haemophilus influenzae*, *Pseudomonas aeruginosa*	*Propionibacterium acnes*, *Nocardia asteroides*
Odontogenic sinusitis	*S. aureus*	*Actinomyces israelii*, gram-negative bacilli, *Peptostreptococcus* spp., *Fusobacterium* spp., pigmented *Prevotella* spp., *Porphyromonas* spp.

CRS (▶ Table 4.4); the number of pathogens involved is also significantly larger and the recovery rate of pathogens is significantly different. Such peculiarities are closely connected to the odontogenic etiology. The odontogenic focus facilitates penetration of the pathogens into the sinus, which is a virtually sterile cavity,[34] and most often acts as a bacterial reservoir that continuously fuels the infection. Dental disease and treatments therefore act as a Trojan horse, allowing into the sinus oral pathogens that normally lack the capacity to cause sinonasal involvement, and sustaining their growth by providing a virtually limitless source from the oral cavity, where these pathogens commonly belong. As these oral pathogens are most often anaerobes (the aerobe to anaerobe ratio in the oral flora ranges from 1:10 to 1:100), it comes as no surprise that anaerobic bacteria play an important role in odontogenic sinusitis and inflammatory SCDDT.

It is important to remember that, as with nonodontogenic CRS, the higher recovery rate of anaerobes in sinusitis may also be related to the long-standing poor drainage and increased intranasal pressure that develop during long periods of unresolved inflammation. A reduction in oxygen tension due to the decreased mucosal blood flow and depressed ciliary action supports the growth of anaerobes.[35,36]

Taking a deeper look into the microbial flora of odontogenic sinusitis, the first thing that comes to the attention is that *S. pneumoniae*, *H. influenzae*, and *M. catarrhalis*—the most frequent isolates in nonodontogenic acute maxillary sinusitis, as previously stated—are virtually absent in odontogenic acute maxillary sinusitis. Another substantial difference from nonodontogenic ARS and CRS is that anaerobic bacteria predominate, with similar isolation rates in both acute and chronic odontogenic sinusitis scenarios. The microbial species described in acute and chronic odontogenic infections are almost invariably anaerobes such as gram-negative bacilli, *Peptostreptococcus* spp., *Fusobacterium* spp., pigmented *Prevotella* spp., and *Porphyromonas* spp., all members of the oropharyngeal flora. All these organisms also predominate in periodontal and endodontal infections.[37,38] *Staphylococcus aureus* is the only aerobe commonly found in odontogenic sinusitis (in about 30% of patients).

It must be pointed out that dental infections, which are generally mixed polymicrobial aerobic and anaerobic bacterial infections, are caused by the same families of oral organisms that are commonly found in inflammatory SCDDT.[37] The association between periapical abscesses and sinusitis is an example of a well-established relationship. When pus aspirates from upper jaw abscesses and their corresponding maxillary sinusitis are compared,[37] a polymicrobial flora is found in all instances, with anaerobes present in all specimens. In this scenario, the predominant isolates are *Prevotella*, *Porphyromonas*, and *Peptostreptococcus* spp. and *Fusobacterium nucleatum*, and microbiological findings are concordant between the periapical abscess and the maxillary sinus flora in all instances, with the exception of few species (*Prevotella gingivalis*, *Streptococcus sanguinis*, and *Streptococcus milleri*) that are not able to thrive well in the sinus cavity.

The lack of consensus between different research groups when comparing odontogenic sinusitis also affects the reported antimicrobial resistance of isolated strains.[39] Nevertheless, some data are universally accepted. The MRSA identification rate can be up to 10%, which is not significantly different from that seen in nonodontogenic CRS. The presence of β-lactamase-positive bacteria, most of them anaerobes, is on the contrary invariably higher than in nonodontogenic ARS and CRS.

Another pathogen, *Actinomyces israelii*, is worthy of mention in this summary. Commonly part of the upper aerodigestive tract flora, *A. israelii* is, however, able to cause potentially devastating infections in most organs. Odontogenic foci may facilitate a mucosal infection, actinomycosis, which manifests with CRS-like symptoms. However, actinomycosis is potentially invasive and is able to spread among the sinuses, invading and destroying bone and cartilage. Luckily, this infection is extremely rare and nonlethal; nevertheless, diagnosis is difficult as it behaves like a neoplasm, and treatment must couple extensive surgical debridement and long-term antibiotic therapy (▶ Fig. 4.1).

4.3.2 Fungi

Nearly 10% of patients who undergo nasal surgery show signs of fungal infection. Focusing only on maxillary sinusitis, this rate rockets to one out of four patients. The somewhat controversial theory originally proposed by Ponikau and colleagues has now been accepted[40]: fungi

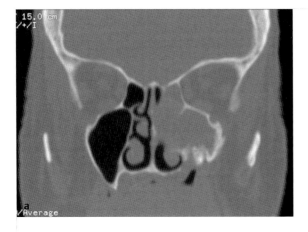
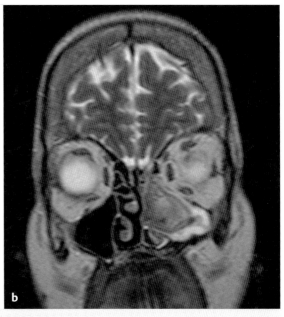

Fig. 4.1 (a) CT scan of a patient with actinomycosis. Note the extensive bone resorption and a partially impacted tooth that presumably acted as the odontogenic focus. (b) T2-weighted MRI of the same patient. Note the composite feature of the image and the clear absence of a signal void, which is typical of fungus ball.

play an indefinite causative role in all chronic sinusitis patients and their presence can be ascertained in more than 95% of patients.

Sinonasal fungal infections represent a diverse class of conditions that range from relatively indolent and common forms, such as paranasal sinus fungus ball, to lethal conditions such as acute fulminant fungal sinusitis, which usually affects only immunocompromised patients.

Since the late 1990s, an improved classification of fungal rhinosinusitis has been developed,[41–43] with strict correlation to the histological patterns found across a range of patients.[44] Briefly, the most commonly accepted classification divides fungal rhinosinusitis into invasive and noninvasive (also called extramucosal) forms, based on the presence or absence, respectively, of microscopic evidence of fungal hyphae within the tissues (mucosa, blood vessels, or bone). The former class is definitely the most prevalent. Classically, it is further divided into allergic fungal sinusitis and fungus ball, along with other non-universally accepted categories such as superficial/saprophytic form, eosinophilic fungal rhinosinusitis, and chronic erosive (noninvasive) sinusitis. Among the invasive forms, three classes are commonly accepted in the literature: granulomatous invasive fungal sinusitis, chronic invasive fungal sinusitis, and acute fulminant fungal sinusitis.

When treating SCDDT patients, otolaryngologists have until now encountered only one kind of fungal rhinosinusitis, namely the paranasal sinus fungus ball. Retrospective reports indicate that 3.7% of patients undergoing surgery for chronic inflammatory nasal conditions have fungus ball, and this rate increases to 28.5% in patients with chronic maxillary sinusitis.[45]

This condition affects women mainly (female to male ratio 2:1) in their sixties, while pediatric patients have not yet been described. The disease is definitely not contagious and spores commonly contaminating the upper airways have been proposed as the source of infection, which is therefore endogenous. There is no known relationship with immune deficiencies (only nonsignificant abnormalities in serum immunoglobulin classes or IgG subclass levels have been demonstrated) and the disease is not associated with pulmonary aspergillosis or pulmonary fungus ball.[46–48]

As for other infectious conditions of the paranasal sinuses, a correlation between anatomical anomalies and fungus ball has been postulated but never demonstrated. Alterations in the nasal septum or conchae occur in up to 15% of patients with paranasal sinus fungus ball, but this is comparable with the general population. No clear relationship between preexisting sinonasal pathology and the incidence of fungus ball has been discovered.

What makes fungus ball so important for SCDDT patients is its high prevalence (1 in 3 patients in Group 3) and its striking relationship with dental procedures. A history of previous dental care procedures—especially dental fillings and, broadly speaking, endodontic procedures—can be established in 56–84% of patients diagnosed with fungus ball and seems to be the only predisposing factor. Several studies have confirmed that endodontic treatments represent a risk factor for maxillary fungus ball.[49,50] The hypothesis is that endodontic materials, which contain zinc oxide–eugenol, promote the growth of *Aspergillus fumigatus*, paralyze cilia, and induce soft tissue hypervascularization and edema, lowering the mucosal defenses.

The fact that there are patients with evidence of a fungus ball and no history of previous dental procedures or diseases, and also patients with nonmaxillary sinus fungus ball (most often sphenoidal fungus ball), suggests that there may be other predisposing factors playing a role in this condition. For example, we report the anecdotal case of a patient with sphenoidal fungus ball who, 7 years before our ENT consultation, had suffered an acute maxillary sinusitis immediately after a root canal procedure, suggesting the sinonasal condition was linked to the dental procedure. Reports such as this—though sporadic—suggest that nonmaxillary sinusitis may also be of odontogenic origin. All patients with fungus ball should therefore undergo specific and accurate history-taking, concentrating on prior dental procedures.

Since the definitive diagnosis of a paranasal sinus fungus ball can often be elusive, deShazo[42] has published five clinicopathological criteria that should be fulfilled in every fungus ball patient: (1) radiological evidence of sinus opacification with or without calcifications; (2) mucopurulent cheesy or claylike materials within the sinus; (3) a dense conglomeration of hyphae (fungus ball) separate from the sinus mucosa; (4) nonspecific chronic inflammation (lymphocytes, plasma cells, eosinophils) of the mucosa without a predominance of eosinophils and without granulomas or allergic mucin; and (5) no histological evidence of fungal invasion of mucosa, blood vessels, or bone visualized microscopically after using special stains for fungus.

Defining the microbiology of fungus ball is as challenging as establishing a definitive diagnosis. When specimens are cultured, negative results are commonplace and only 23–50% of cultures yield fungal growth.[51] One reason may be the low viability of fungal cells in the fungus ball. Most specimens yield positive results for *Aspergillus* spp. (93% of positive cultures identified *Aspergillus fumigatus* according to Dufour et al[47]). *Aspergillus fumigatus* is not an infective agent: on the contrary it is found ubiquitously in the soil, where it plays a saprophytic role growing on decomposing vegetable material. Its sporulated conidia are so small that they can penetrate both nasal sinuses and lung alveoli. If we consider that *Aspergillus* spp. are commonly eliminated effortlessly every day by the innate immune system of the majority of humans, the role of predisposing factors appears even more relevant. Occasionally specimens yield positive results for other fungi, such as *Scedosporium apiospermum* (*Pseudallescheria apiosperma*), *Aspergillus flavus, niger*, or *terreus*, and *Pleurophomopsis lignicola*.

Some authors report in case series of nonodontogenic fungus ball a potentially important role for fungi of the genus *Mucor*.[34,52] However, the identification of *Mucor* species is based only on morphology on histological slides or immunohistochemical staining, and this fungus has never been cultured from patients with fungus ball. Therefore, in these patients, the true identity of the involved fungus is questionable. The role for *Mucor*-like species in odontogenic sinusitis has yet to be assessed.

Due to the relatively poor yield of fungal culture, even in expert hands, this technique has only a speculative role; correct identification of the causative fungal species is not required to properly treat fungus balls in SCDDT patients. Surgery is usually adequate treatment, without antimycotic drugs. On the contrary, definitive microscopic examination is mandatory in patients with suspected tissue invasion. If confirmed, a diagnosis of SCDDT should be ruled out and identification of the responsible fungus by culture may be crucial in selecting the necessary antimycotic treatment.

To conclude this brief discussion on fungus balls, it must be pointed out that sinonasal fungus ball, despite lacking infective potential per se, hosts a number of infectious and diverse bacterial microorganisms, comparable to those seen in bacterial SCDDT. The presence of several species can be closely related to a change in the sinonasal environment linked to the odontogenic focus. In this complex relationship we have yet to discover whether fungi and bacterial species show a kind of symbiotic behavior that amplifies their infective capabilities. We therefore propose that postsurgical antibiotic therapy should become mandatory in managing these patients, in marked contrast to those authors who advocate surgical therapy alone.

Key Points

- The oral microbiome plays a major role in odontogenic sinusitis and SCDDT. Dental conditions and dental procedures act as a "Trojan horse" allowing a massive transfer of pathogens into the sinonasal cavities.
- The oral ecosystem is home to various human symbionts, including viruses, protozoa, fungi, archaea, and bacteria. Oral microbes live primarily as biofilms. Biofilms allow bacteria to live in a protected nutrient-rich milieu.
- The oral microbiota is known to be a reservoir for infection at other body sites.
- Anaerobic bacteria have a predominant role in odontogenic sinusitis and inflammatory SCDDT. The microbial species described in acute and chronic odontogenic infections are almost invariably anaerobes such as gram-negative bacilli, *Peptostreptococcus* spp., *Fusobacterium* spp., pigmented *Prevotella* spp., and *Porphyromonas* spp., all members of the oropharyngeal flora.

- When treating SCDDT patients, otolaryngologists at present encounter only one kind of fungal rhinosinusitis, namely paranasal sinus fungus ball. Fungus ball, despite being devoid of infective potential per se, hosts a number of infectious and diverse bacterial microorganisms comparable to those seen in bacterial SCDDT.

References

[1] Fokkens WJ, Lund VJ, Mullol J et al. EPOS 2012: European position paper on rhinosinusitis and nasal polyps 2012. A summary for otorhinolaryngologists. Rhinology 2012; 50: 1–12

[2] Dewhirst FE, Chen T, Izard J et al. The human oral microbiome. J Bacteriol 2010; 192: 5002–5017

[3] Wade WG. The oral microbiome in health and disease. Pharmacol Res 2013; 69: 137–143

[4] Slots J, Slots H. Bacterial and viral pathogens in saliva: disease relationship and infectious risk. Periodontol 2000 2011; 55: 48–69

[5] Pride DT, Salzman J, Haynes M et al. Evidence of a robust resident bacteriophage population revealed through analysis of the human salivary virome. ISME J 2012; 6: 915–926

[6] Ghannoum MA, Jurevic RJ, Mukherjee PK et al. Characterization of the oral fungal microbiome (mycobiome) in healthy individuals. PLoS Pathog 2010; 6: e1000713

[7] Human Microbiome Project Consortium. Structure, function and diversity of the healthy human microbiome. Nature 2012; 486: 207–214

[8] Segata N, Haake SK, Mannon P et al. Composition of the adult digestive tract bacterial microbiome based on seven mouth surfaces, tonsils, throat and stool samples. Genome Biol 2012; 13: R42

[9] Zaura E, Keijser BJ, Huse SM, Crielaard W. Defining the healthy "core microbiome" of oral microbial communities. BMC Microbiol 2009; 9: 259

[10] Lazarevic V, Whiteson K, Hernandez D, François P, Schrenzel J. Study of inter- and intra-individual variations in the salivary microbiota. BMC Genomics 2010; 11: 523

[11] Nasidze I, Li J, Quinque D, Tang K, Stoneking M. Global diversity in the human salivary microbiome. Genome Res 2009; 19: 636–643

[12] Hamady M, Knight R. Microbial community profiling for human microbiome projects: Tools, techniques, and challenges. Genome Res 2009; 19: 1141–1152

[13] Rothberg JM, Hinz W, Rearick TM et al. An integrated semiconductor device enabling non-optical genome sequencing. Nature 2011; 475: 348–352

[14] Dassi E, Ballarini A, Covello G et al. HTM-CMB2013. Enhanced microbial diversity in the saliva microbiome induced by short-term probiotic intake revealed by 16S rRNA sequencing on the IonTorrent PGM platform. J Biotechnol 2014; 190: 30–39

[15] Jünemann S, Prior K, Szczepanowski R et al. Bacterial community shift in treated periodontitis patients revealed by ion torrent 16S rRNA gene amplicon sequencing. PLoS ONE 2012; 7: e41606

[16] Takahashi N, Nyvad B. The role of bacteria in the caries process: ecological perspectives. J Dent Res 2011; 90: 294–303

[17] Downes J, Mantzourani M, Beighton D et al. Scardovia wiggsiae sp. nov., isolated from the human oral cavity and clinical material, and emended descriptions of the genus Scardovia and Scardovia inopinata. Int J Syst Evol Microbiol 2011; 61: 25–29

[18] Tanner AC, Kent RL Jr, Holgerson PL et al. Microbiota of severe early childhood caries before and after therapy. J Dent Res 2011; 90: 1298–1305

[19] Kumar PS, Mason MR, Janel Y. Biofilms in periodontal health and disease. In: Jakubovics NS, Palmer RJ Jr, eds. Oral Microbial Ecology:

Current Research and New Perspectives. Norfolk, UK: Caister Academic Press; 2013:153–166

[20] Ahn J, Chen CY, Hayes RB. Oral microbiome and oral and gastrointestinal cancer risk. Cancer Causes Control 2012; 23: 399–404

[21] Farrell JJ, Zhang L, Zhou H et al. Variations of oral microbiota are associated with pancreatic diseases including pancreatic cancer. Gut 2012; 61: 582–588

[22] Huang S, Yang F, Zeng X et al. Preliminary characterization of the oral microbiota of Chinese adults with and without gingivitis. BMC Oral Health 2011; 11: 33

[23] Yang F, Zeng X, Ning K et al. Saliva microbiomes distinguish caries-active from healthy human populations. ISME J 2012; 6: 1–10

[24] Han YW, Wang X. Mobile microbiome: oral bacteria in extra-oral infections and inflammation. J Dent Res 2013; 92: 485–491

[25] Coelho ED, Arrais JP, Matos S et al. Computational prediction of the human-microbial oral interactome. BMC Syst Biol 2014; 8: 24

[26] Mehra P, Jeong D. Maxillary sinusitis of odontogenic origin. Curr Infect Dis Rep 2008; 10: 205–210

[27] Brook I. The role of anaerobic bacteria in sinusitis. Anaerobe 2006; 12: 5–12

[28] Brook I. Recovery of aerobic and anaerobic bacteria in sinus fungal ball. Otolaryngol Head Neck Surg 2011; 145: 851–852

[29] Jousimies-Somer HR, Savolainen S, Ylikoski JS. Bacteriological findings of acute maxillary sinusitis in young adults. J Clin Microbiol 1988; 26: 1919–1925

[30] Kalcioglu MT, Durmaz B, Aktas E, Ozturan O, Durmaz R. Bacteriology of chronic maxillary sinusitis and normal maxillary sinuses: using culture and multiplex polymerase chain reaction. Am J Rhinol 2003; 17: 143–147

[31] Nord CE. The role of anaerobic bacteria in recurrent episodes of sinusitis and tonsillitis. Clin Infect Dis 1995; 20: 1512–1524

[32] Patel NA, Ferguson BJ. Odontogenic sinusitis: an ancient but underappreciated cause of maxillary sinusitis. Curr Opin Otolaryngol Head Neck Surg 2012; 20: 24–28

[33] Brook I. Sinusitis of odontogenic origin. Otolaryngol Head Neck Surg 2006; 135: 349–355

[34] Robey AB, O'Brien EK, Richardson BE, Baker JJ, Poage DP, Leopold DA. The changing face of paranasal sinus fungus balls. Ann Otol Rhinol Laryngol 2009; 118: 500–505

[35] Aust R, Stierna P, Drettner B. Basic experimental studies of ostial patency and local metabolic environment of the maxillary sinus. Acta Otolaryngol Suppl 1994; 515: 7–10, discussion 11

[36] Carenfelt C. Pathogenesis of sinus empyema. Ann Otol Rhinol Laryngol 1979; 88: 16–20

[37] Brook I. Microbiology and management of endodontic infections in children. J Clin Pediatr Dent 2003; 28: 13–17

[38] Kuriyama T, Williams DW, Yanagisawa M et al. Antimicrobial susceptibility of 800 anaerobic isolates from patients with dentoalveolar infection to 13 oral antibiotics. Oral Microbiol Immunol 2007; 22: 285–288

[39] Puglisi S, Privitera S, Maiolino L et al. Bacteriological findings and antimicrobial resistance in odontogenic and non-odontogenic chronic maxillary sinusitis. J Med Microbiol 2011; 60: 1353–1359

[40] Ponikau JU, Sherris DA, Kern EB et al. The diagnosis and incidence of allergic fungal sinusitis. Mayo Clin Proc 1999; 74: 877–884

[41] Chakrabarti A, Denning DW, Ferguson BJ et al. Fungal rhinosinusitis: a categorization and definitional schema addressing current controversies. Laryngoscope 2009; 119: 1809–1818

[42] deShazo RD, O'Brien M, Chapin K, Soto-Aguilar M, Gardner L. Swain R. A new classification and diagnostic criteria for invasive fungal sinusitis. Arch Otolaryngol Head Neck Surg 1997; 123: 1181–1188

[43] Uri N, Cohen-Kerem R, Elmalah I, Doweck I, Greenberg E. Classification of fungal sinusitis in immunocompetent patients. Otolaryngol Head Neck Surg 2003; 129: 372–378

[44] Granville L, Chirala M, Cernoch P, Ostrowski M, Truong LD. Fungal sinusitis: histologic spectrum and correlation with culture. Hum Pathol 2004; 35: 474–481

[45] Ferreiro JA, Carlson BA, Cody DT III. Paranasal sinus fungus balls. Head Neck 1997; 19: 481–486

[46] Dufour X, Kauffmann-Lacroix C, Ferrie J-C et al. Paranasal sinus fungus ball and surgery: a review of 175 cases. Rhinology 2005; 43: 34–39

[47] Dufour X, Kauffmann-Lacroix C, Ferrie JC, Goujon JM, Rodier MH, Klossek JM. Paranasal sinus fungus ball: epidemiology, clinical features and diagnosis. A retrospective analysis of 173 cases from a single medical center in France, 1989–2002. Med Mycol 2006; 44: 61–67

[48] Grosjean P, Weber R. Fungus balls of the paranasal sinuses: a review. Eur Arch Otorhinolaryngol 2007; 264: 461–470

[49] Mensi M, Piccioni M, Marsili F, Nicolai P, Sapelli PL, Latronico N. Risk of maxillary fungus ball in patients with endodontic treatment on maxillary teeth: a case-control study. Oral Surg Oral Med Oral Pathol Oral Radiol Endod 2007; 103: 433–436

[50] Park GY, Kim HY, Min J-Y, Dhong HJ, Chung SK. Endodontic treatment: a significant risk factor for the development of maxillary fungal ball. Clin Exp Otorhinolaryngol 2010; 3: 136–140

[51] Ferguson BJ. Fungus balls of the paranasal sinuses. Otolaryngol Clin North Am 2000; 33: 389–398

[52] Ma L, Xu R, Shi J et al. Identification of fungi in fungal ball sinusitis: comparison between MUC5B immunohistochemical and Grocott methenamine silver staining. Acta Otolaryngol 2013; 133: 1181–1187

Chapter 5

Medical Treatment of Odontogenic Sinusitis

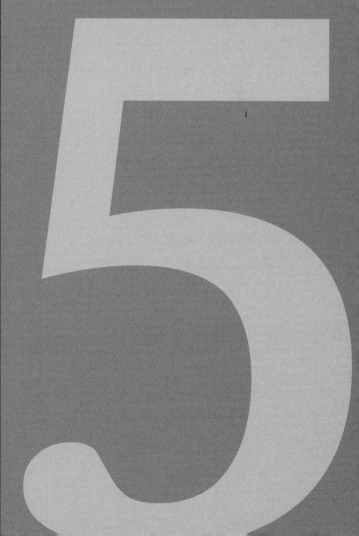

5 Medical Treatment of Odontogenic Sinusitis

Antonella D'Arminio-Monforte, Teresa Bini, Alberto Scotti, Alberto Maria Saibene, Carlotta Pipolo

Contents Overview

This chapter will deal with the medical therapy of odontogenic sinusitis. Both systemic therapy and local therapy will be discussed, along with current evidence on the subject. The chapter focuses first on treating acute onset odontogenic sinusitis and secondly on the correct perioperative and postoperative treatment of patients with sinonasal complications of dental disease or treatment (SCDDT). Quick reference tables of treatment recommendations are provided.

5.1 Introduction

Odontogenic sinusitis is a well-known condition, accounting for 10 to 12% of patients with maxillary sinusitis. Medical therapy for this specific type of sinusitis is still based on best practice and guidelines for nonodontogenic sinusitis, as no shared international recommendations are available.[1] However, when tackling the acute and chronic infectious responses to dental pathologies and complications related to oral implants and maxillary sinus grafting, otolaryngologists and oral surgeons must constantly remind themselves of the different etiology and pathophysiology compared with nonodontogenic sinusitis.[2] Furthermore, medical therapy alone will have limited success, as the underlying dental cause will often need to be addressed surgically. Nevertheless, proper and timely treatment of acute SCDDT can spare the patient costly and lengthy surgical procedures and lead to a quick recovery.

Starting from the most widely recognized nonodontogenic acute and chronic sinusitis treatment guidelines and focusing in particular on the peculiar features of SCDDT, the following sections will provide detailed information and algorithms regarding antibiotic and topical therapy, both during the acute phase and after surgical treatment.

5.2 Treatment of Acute Odontogenic Sinusitis

5.2.1 Treatment of the Odontogenic Focus

Most acute SCDDT stem from an easily recognizable odontogenic/dental focus: dental abscesses, superinfected periapical granulomas, destructive caries, recently placed oral implants, and grafting materials used for maxillary reconstruction or sinus grafting to allow immediate or subsequent implant placement are common sources of acute SCDDT.

Whenever an odontogenic focus is identified, this should be the primary target for treatment. Elimination of the odontogenic focus means that the infection loses its primary bacterial reservoir and becomes more easily controllable with systemic and local therapy, without the need for further nasal surgical procedures. Furthermore, acting on the primary odontogenic source of infection allows the biofilm, which normally protects oral pathogens from antibiotic treatment, to be partially destroyed.

The complete treatment of these odontogenic foci is far too wide a subject to be comprehensively covered in this textbook, although some of the most important techniques are briefly covered in Chapter 6 (p.84). The oral surgeon should bear in mind that common treatments for these conditions (endodontics, extractions, alveolar curettage, and so on) also retain their usefulness in patients with acute SCDDT and should be coupled with the correct systemic and local treatment, as described in later sections of this chapter.

As far as SCDDT are concerned, there are three main elements that the oral surgeon or the consulting otolaryngologist should bear in mind when evaluating the patient:

- Odontogenic foci that are displaced into the sinuses (whether iatrogenically or not) are generally not amenable to treatment without employing surgical techniques, whether endoscopic or conventional. Such patients should therefore avoid purely medical treatment and are candidates for proper surgical treatment. For further details, please refer to Chapter 6 (p.84).
- When treating acute sinusitis following maxillary sinus grafting, there is a chance to stop the infective process with proper antibiotic therapy and, possibly, graft removal only if Schneider's membrane has not been damaged.[3] If the infected grafting material bypasses Schneider's membrane, there are few chances to treat the resulting sinusitis without a surgical procedure, since the grafting material has to be surgically removed from the whole sinus. If the infected graft remains under Schneider's membrane, it is possible to remove the infection focus via the same surgical access used for the maxillary sinus grafting procedure.
- When treating the odontogenic focus, the oral surgeon should remember that oroantral communications opened during acute sinusitis are virtually impossible to close, even if the proper systemic treatment is administered to the patient. Should an oroantral communication open, the purulent secretions should be drained gently from the maxillary sinus in order to lower endosinusal pressure and bacterial load, and the communication should be closed with the aid of completely tension-free local flaps.

5.2.2 Antibiotic Treatment

Based on microbiology findings, as seen in Chapter 4 (p. 66), the bacterial pathogens implicated in odontogenic sinusitis are those most commonly identified in the normal oral and oropharyngeal flora. In particular, these isolates include both aerobic and anaerobic bacteria: the predominant aerobes are alpha-hemolytic streptococci, microaerophilic streptococci, and *Staphylococcus aureus*, together with anaerobic bacteria, such as *Peptostreptococcus* spp., *Prevotella melaninogenica*, and *Fusobacterium*.[4,5] Therefore, whenever possible, a nasal swab or aspiration of sinus content through nasal or sinus endoscopy should support a correct etiological diagnosis; samples should be collected in both aerobic and anaerobic media.

First-line empiric therapy for acute odontogenic sinusitis of all origins (dental/implant/grafting) should include a 2-week course of amoxicillin/clavulanate (875/125 mg orally q8h) or doxycycline (100 mg orally q12h) or trimethoprim/sulfamethoxazole (800/160 mg orally q8h). Second-line therapy should include a 2-week course of levofloxacin (500–750 mg orally q24h) or ciprofloxacin (500 mg orally q12h) or clarithromycin (500 mg orally q12h). Therapy should be modified according to the results of microbiological testing and individual intolerance.[6] See ▸ Table 5.1 for a quick reference.

In patients with chronic odontogenic sinusitis (symptoms of sinusitis lasting more than 12 weeks) and/or a second acute episode, the same medical management, including culture whenever possible and a 3- to 4-week course of antibiotic therapy, is recommended. In this particular context, long-term antibiotic therapy has been reported to improve symptoms in chronic odontogenic sinusitis refractive to corticosteroid therapy.[6–9]

In 2008, a meta-analysis of randomized trials compared ciprofloxacin to amoxicillin/clavulanate in acute sinusitis showed no significant difference in symptom improvement between the two antibiotics,[10] although it should be noted that these data were extracted from the records of classic "rhinogenic" sinusitis patients.

5.2.3 Systemic Support Treatment

Supporting medical therapies are mostly based on oral corticosteroids. This class of drugs has been deemed useful for acute nonodontogenic sinusitis in addition to antibiotic therapies and is effective for short-term relief of symptoms (e.g., headache, facial pain, nasal decongestion). We recommend 8 mg methylprednisolone 3 times daily for 5 days. Oral antihistamines are not recommended.

5.2.4 Local Treatment

Topic nasal treatments in acute and chronic rhinosinusitis represent a field of intense debate among rhinologists and infectious disease specialists. Most topical nasal treatments do not have a sound scientific basis, but their use is an important part of everyday best practice, whether in the acute, chronic, or postsurgical scenarios.

As for local treatment of other features of odontogenic sinusitis, universally recognized guidelines are still not available; most data in the literature are based on small case series, and prospective randomized studies are completely lacking.

It should also be noted that topical therapy in acute odontogenic sinusitis must take into account the role of strict oral hygiene, especially after local oral procedures.

In order to promote the highest rates of success, local treatment should be coupled with the correct systemic antibiotic and steroid treatment, described in Sections 5.2.2 (p. 77) and 5.2.3 (p. 77). The choice of which local treatments to combine with these is of course up to the surgeon, although a guide based on our best practice is given in ▸ Table 5.2 for reference.

Nasal Treatments

Nasal lavages

Nasal lavages are almost universally recommended in acute rhinosinusitis,[11,12] as they help to clear the mucopurulent secretions from the nasal cavities without damaging the nasal mucosa. This is especially important in acute rhinosinusitis given the impaired ciliary movement

Table 5.1 Recommended antibiotic treatment for acute chronic odontogenic sinusitis and acute exacerbations of chronic odontogenic sinusitis

First line: acute odontogenic sinusitis (14-day course)	Amoxicillin/clavulanate (875/125 mg orally q8h)	Doxycycline (100 mg orally q12h)	Trimethoprim/sulfamethoxazole (800/160 mg orally q8h)
Second line: acute odontogenic sinusitis (14-day course)	Levofloxacin (500–750 mg orally q24h)	Ciprofloxacin (500 mg orally q12h)	Clarithromycin (500 mg orally q12h)
Chronic odontogenic sinusitis/second episode (21–28 days)	After swab or aspirate same as above if indicated	After swab or aspirate same as above if indicated	After swab or aspirate same as above if indicated

Table 5.2 Topical treatments in acute SCDDT

Treatment	Recommendation	Treatment suggestion
Nasal lavages	Yes	Saline lavages 3–4 times a day for 1 month, preferably with compressible douching system
Topical steroids	Yes	Fluticasone furoate 27.5 µg, 2 puffs daily in each nostril for 1 month
Antihistamines	No	
Nasal decongestants	Yes (no published evidence)	Naphazoline, 2 puffs in each nostril 3 times a day for no more than 5 days
Topical antibiotics	No	
Mouth rinses	Yes (if recent oral surgical procedure)	Chlorhexidine 0.2% oral rinse, 3 times a day for 7–10 days

caused by mucosal edema and inflammation. In order to minimize damage to the nasal mucosa, most guidelines suggest using saline solutions, while some authors advocate the use of additives such as baby shampoo,[13] sodium hypochlorite,[14] or xylitol[15] in the saline. The effects of adding antibiotics to lavages are controversial, while adding antifungals is definitely pointless.[16,17] Some controversy still remains concerning the type of device that should be used for nasal lavages, given that most devices are to a certain extent beneficial. Campos et al performed an in vitro comparison of nasal douching systems, demonstrating the theoretical superiority of the compressible douching system. Nasal lavages should be performed no less than 3 times a day.

Topical steroids

Topical steroids have a proven and widely recognized beneficial effect in treating acute rhinosinusitis. Cochrane reviews and EPOS guidelines[12,19] recommend the use of topical mometasone furoate or fluticasone furoate during the acute phase of rhinosinusitis. The anti-inflammatory and anti-edema effects of these drugs far outweigh the mild local immune suppression. Topical steroids in odontogenic sinusitis represent first-line treatment aimed at enhancing the patency of the ostiomeatal complex and allowing maxillary sinus drainage.

Antihistamines

Although topical antihistamine drugs are suggested as ancillary therapy during acute rhinosinusitis,[12] they have no role in acute odontogenic sinusitis, as patients suffer in virtually all cases from bacterial infections.

Nasal decongestants

Nasal decongestants have a potential detrimental effect on the nasal mucosa due to the risks of rebound congestion and *rhinitis medicamentosa*.[20] Furthermore, nasal decongestants have no proven role in the treatment of acute rhinosinusitis. Nevertheless, best practice in odontogenic sinusitis suggests using brief "shock courses" of nasal decongestants (e.g., naphazoline) in order to force open the blockade of the ostiomeatal complex and restore the maxillary sinus drainage. If the course of nasal decongestants (usually 2 puffs in each nostril 3 times a day for no more than 5 days) succeeds in restoring maxillary sinus drainage, the rise in oxygen levels inside the sinus is usually enough to halt the growth of anaerobes, which are known to have an important role in the development of chronic rhinosinusitis.

Topical antibiotics

Topical antibiotics, delivered as ointments or creams, have no role in acute rhinosinusitis, since the drug delivery rates are far too low inside the sinuses.

Oral Treatments

Mouth rinses

There is no evidence on the role of mouth rinses and oral hygiene in treating odontogenic infections, especially sinonasal infections. Nevertheless, several studies support the efficacy of rinses in treating bacterial diseases of the mouth, such as caries,[21] and in lowering bacteremia after oral surgery procedures.[22] Furthermore, the use of mouth rinses is considered best practice in the majority of oral surgery procedures, despite the lack of strong evidence. All evidence in the literature unanimously supports the use of mouth rinses containing chlorhexidine, because of its known wide-spectrum activity. Commercially available alcohol-based chlorhexidine solutions contain 0.12 to 0.2% chlorhexidine, although several studies have demonstrated the tolerability and efficacy of 0.3% chlorhexidine solutions.[23] There is no literature available on the use of mouth rinses in SCDDT. However, if we combine the existing data with current best practice, there is strong support for using 0.2% chlorhexidine mouth rinses 3 or 4 times a day whenever an acute

SCDDT occurs, specifically when the complication follows implant insertion, maxillary sinus grafting, or dental extraction, with or without oroantral communication. Since the dental focus acts as a "Trojan horse" by inoculating pathogens into the maxillary sinus, lowering the bacterial load at the primary infection site is of paramount importance when treating acute SCDDT.

Last but not least, the oral surgeon should always recommend to patients suffering from acute SCDDT who have undergone any recent dental procedures that they use the best possible oral hygiene. Simply cleaning teeth with an ordinary toothbrush is the first-line procedure to ensure prompt healing, despite often being neglected or intentionally avoided by patients who have undergone oral surgery.

5.3 Perioperative Medical Care of Odontogenic Sinusitis

When dealing surgically with chronic rhinosinusitis, even the best procedure has a high risk of failure if the patient is not supported and instructed in the best techniques for nasal care. Even if there is no ultimate consensus on postoperative treatments for patients undergoing endoscopic sinus surgery, some local therapies are generally accepted and encouraged by international societies.[12]

Systemic therapy is a matter of intense debate, since there is no decisive evidence on the role of antibiotic therapy during postoperative care for chronic rhinosinusitis patients. Not surprisingly, when dealing surgically with odontogenic sinusitis and SCDDT, antibiotic therapy becomes pivotal in the correct treatment of patients, as a result of the peculiar role oral pathogens, anaerobes, and biofilms play in this condition. Therefore long-term specific antibiotic therapy should always be coupled with local therapies after surgical treatment of patients with inflammatory SCDDT. The correct antibiotic regimen is a great help in dealing with the frequent acute exacerbations of chronic SCDDT, which may be present at the time of surgery, thereby raising the postoperative complication rate. Of course, when dealing with noninflammatory SCDDT such as displaced implants, there is no need for systemic therapies, despite local therapies retaining an extremely important role in the healing of the nasal mucosa.

5.3.1 Systemic Therapy

Cultures from the sinus cavity either during sinus endoscopy or at a later stage, during sinus surgery, are highly recommended in order to identify the flora involved; samples should be collected in both aerobic and anaerobic media.

In contrast to perioperative medical treatment in classic sinusitis, we advocate the use of antibiotic therapy before and after surgery. This is based on our experience and the different nature of odontogenic sinusitis, with abundant purulent secretion and/or foreign bodies present at the time of surgery. Antibiotic therapy should start, depending on the extent of infection, 1 week or 1 day before surgery and continue for up to 14 to 21 days in order to sterilize the affected area. The optimum duration of antibiotic therapy after surgery has not yet been defined and may depend upon the severity of the initial infection and antibiotic resistance, as in many cases the patient undergoing surgical intervention has already been given multiple courses of antibiotics by their dentist, starting at the time of the first manifestation of disease. In this situation, resistant bacteria may have been selected by antibiotic underdosage or underdiffusion: antibiotics may not have reached the seriously infected area because of the purulent secretion. In any case, an empiric therapy should be started before surgery and could be changed on the basis of the antibiogram, once available.

On the basis of these considerations, at the time of surgical intervention we can distinguish two different scenarios: a patient with untreated odontogenic sinusitis and a patient with odontogenic sinusitis previously treated with several lines of antibiotic therapy.

In general, amoxicillin/clavulanate remains the first choice for uncomplicated odontogenic sinusitis, but the growing prevalence of resistant strains limits its use.

The recommendations for initial empiric therapy, as shown in ▶ Table 5.3, are as follows:
- First-line empiric therapy (in patients with untreated odontogenic sinusitis): amoxicillin/clavulanate (875/125 mg orally q8h)
- Experienced empiric therapy (in patients with previously treated odontogenic sinusitis): levofloxacin (500–750 mg q24h) or trimethoprim/sulfamethoxazole (800/160 mg q8h).

In patients with severe disease, a parenteral regimen should be considered:
- Piperacillin/tazobactam (4.5 g IV q6h) plus vancomycin (1 g load followed by 500 mg q6h),
- Or clindamycin (600 mg IV q8h), plus ceftriaxone (2 g IV q24h),
- Or carbapenem (imipenem 500 mg IV q6h, or meropenem 1 g IV q8h).

Vancomycin should be added in patients with severe disease involving suspected penicillin-resistant organisms.

5.3.2 Local Therapy

Local therapy has a fundamental and universally recognized postoperative role in patients who have undergone endoscopic sinus surgery. Even in the context of minimal invasiveness, the surgical maneuvers result in mucosal

Table 5.3 Recommended perioperative antibiotic treatment

First line: perioperative empiric treatment	Amoxicillin/clavulanate (875/125 mg orally q8h)		
Experienced empiric therapy (in patients with previously treated odontogenic sinusitis)	Levofloxacin (500–750 mg orally q24h)	Trimethoprim/sulfamethoxazole (800/160 mg orally q8h)	
In severe/complicated disease (Add vancomycin in patients with suspected penicillin-resistant organisms)	Piperacillin/tazobactam (4.5 g IV q6h) plus vancomycin (1 g load followed by 500 mg q6h)	Clindamycin (600 mg IV q8h), plus ceftriaxone (2 g IV q24h)	Carbapenem-class antibiotics (imipenem 500 mg IV q6h, or meropenem 1 g IV q8h)

Table 5.4 Postoperative topical treatments in SCDDT

Treatment	Recommendation	Treatment suggestion
Nasal lavages (with or without hyaluronate)	Yes	Saline lavages 3–4 times a day for 1 month, preferably with compressible douching system OR Saline lavages 3–4 times a day for 1 month, preferably with compressible douching system, plus sodium hyaluronate 9 mg twice daily
Topical steroids	Yes (in inflammatory SCDDT)	Fluticasone furoate 27.5 µg, 2 puffs daily in each nostril for 1 month
Antihistamines	No	
Nasal decongestants	No	
Topical antibiotics	Yes, especially with *Staphylococcus aureus* infections	Mupirocin ointment, 3 times a day for 2 weeks
Mouth rinses	Yes (if oral or combined surgical procedure)	Chlorhexidine 0.2% oral rinse, 3 times a day for 7–10 days

damage and, therefore, inflammation that is scarcely distinguishable from an acute sinusitis. The mucosal swelling slows down the healing process and patient recovery, and threatens the newly restored sinusal patency with the development of scar tissue and synechiae.

Therefore, patients who have undergone endoscopic sinus surgery should follow local therapy protocols similar to those for patients with acute SCDDT, with few exceptions. These protocols are listed in ▶ Table 5.4 for quick reference.

The rationale for lavages, topical steroids, and mouth rinses is the same as for acute rhinosinusitis. Adding hyaluronate to nasal lavages postoperatively appears to speed up the recovery of patients and mucosal healing.[24,25]

Antihistamine drugs still have no role and nasal decongestants should be avoided in case they cause further damage to the nasal mucosa.

In contrast to acute rhinosinusitis, patients with surgically treated chronic/recurrent odontogenic sinusitis

benefit from the use of topical intranasal mupirocin cream (q8h), especially when cultures yield positive results for *S. aureus*.

5.3.3 Fungus Ball

The final diagnosis of paranasal sinus fungus ball can be made only intra- or postoperatively: despite some suggestive radiological signs, only findings of a brownish mass inside the sinus and histological identification of extramucosal hyphae can confirm the presence of a fungus ball, as described in Chapters 2 (p. 16) and 4 (p. 66). Furthermore, though the clinical presentation of fungus ball is usually enough to distinguish these mycoses from invasive forms, histological lack of intramucosal involvement is required for final diagnosis. Therefore we will briefly discuss only the postoperative medical management of patients with fungus balls, since there is no need or scope for any presurgical therapy.

Paranasal fungus ball is an extramucosal fungal proliferation, usually involving the maxillary or sphenoid sinuses; multiple localizations are rare. It is mostly caused by *Aspergillus* spp.; other fungi occasionally cultured are *Scedosporium apiospermum*, *Aspergillus flavus*, *niger*, or *terrus*, and *Pleurophomopsis lignicola*. Please refer to Chapter 4 (p. 66) for more details. It has been described that fungal rhinosinusitis, when including all subgroups of fungal involvement, is encountered in 10 to 12% of patients undergoing sinus surgery[26] and case series state that the prevalence of fungus ball at time of surgery is around 4%.[27]

Cultures are frequently negative and this is probably related to the poor viability of the fungal elements in the fungus ball. The mucosa shows a nonspecific inflammation, in which plasma cells and lymphocytes are predominant. A fungus ball should be suspected in any patient with recurrent or refractory unilateral sinusitis. Definitive diagnosis is made by the characteristic macroscopic image and by histopathological examination. Macroscopically, the fungus ball is characterized by friable material; microscopically it is represented by an aggregate of hyphae.

Regarding treatment, in patients with suspected fungus ball the indication of surgical treatment is mandatory. After surgery, no local or systemic antimycotic treatment is recommended, as surgery achieves healing in almost 100% of patients without recurrence. Antibiotic treatment is, nevertheless, indicated in all patients, as bacterial superinfections are present in virtually all paranasal sinus fungus balls, as described in Chapter 5 (p. 76).

Key Points

- Proper and timely treatment of acute odontogenic sinusitis and SCDDT may lead to patient recovery even without additional surgical treatments.
- Prompt recognition of the dental focus is pivotal in treating acute SCDDT.
- Long-term antibiotic treatment has a fundamental role, especially in chronic odontogenic rhinosinusitis, and should be culture-driven whenever possible, both in the acute setting and postoperatively.
- Patient treatment cannot be considered complete without the addition of local ancillary therapies, which facilitate more rapid healing and recovery, both in the acute setting and postoperatively.
- Fungus ball does not require antifungal treatment, despite requiring antibiotic therapy for the bacterial superinfection.

References

[1] Felisati G, Chiapasco M, Lozza P et al. Sinonasal complications resulting from dental treatment: outcome-oriented proposal of classification and surgical protocol. Am J Rhinol Allergy 2013; 27: e101–e106

[2] Arias-Irimia O, Barona-Dorado C, Santos-Marino JA, Martínez-Rodriguez N, Martínez-González JM. Meta-analysis of the etiology of odontogenic maxillary sinusitis. Med Oral Patol Oral Cir Bucal 2010; 15: e70–e73

[3] Testori T, Drago L, Wallace SS et al. Prevention and treatment of postoperative infections after sinus elevation surgery: clinical consensus and recommendations. Int J Dent 2012; 2012: 365809Epub2012Aug9

[4] Brook I. Sinusitis of odontogenic origin. Otolaryngol Head Neck Surg 2006; 135: 349–355 Review

[5] Brook I. The role of anaerobic bacteria in sinusitis. Anaerobe 2006; 12: 5–12

[6] Farmahan S, Tuopar D, Ameerally PJ, Kotecha R, Sisodia B. Microbiological examination and antibiotic sensitivity of infections in the head and neck. Has anything changed? Br J Oral Maxillofac Surg 2014; 52: 632–635

[7] Adelson RT, Adappa ND. What is the proper role of oral antibiotics in the treatment of patients with chronic sinusitis? Curr Opin Otolaryngol Head Neck Surg 2013; 21: 61–68

[8] Chen YW, Huang CC, Chang PH et al. The characteristics and new treatment paradigm of dental implant-related chronic rhinosinusitis. Am J Rhinol Allergy 2013; 27: 237–244

[9] Mandal R, Patel N, Ferguson BJ. Role of antibiotics in sinusitis. Curr Opin Infect Dis 2012; 25: 183–192

[10] Karageorgopoulos DE, Giannopoulou KP, Grammatikos AP, Dimopoulos G, Falagas ME. Fluoroquinolones compared with beta-lactam antibiotics for the treatment of acute bacterial sinusitis: a meta-analysis of randomized controlled trials. CMAJ 2008; 178: 845–854

[11] Chow AW, Benninger MS, Brook I et al. Infectious Diseases Society of America. IDSA clinical practice guideline for acute bacterial rhinosinusitis in children and adults. Clin Infect Dis 2012; 54: e72–e112

[12] Fokkens WJ, Lund VJ, Mullol J et al. EPOS 2012: European position paper on rhinosinusitis and nasal polyps 2012. A summary for otorhinolaryngologists. Rhinology 2012; 50: 1–12

[13] Rosen PL, Palmer JN, O'Malley BW Jr, Cohen NA. Surfactants in the management of rhinopathologies. Am J Rhinol Allergy 2013; 27: 177–180

[14] Raza T, Elsherif HS, Zulianello L, Plouin-Gaudon I, Landis BN, Lacroix JS. Nasal lavage with sodium hypochlorite solution in Staphylococcus aureus persistent rhinosinusitis. Rhinology 2008; 46: 15–22

[15] Weissman JD, Fernandez F, Hwang PH. Xylitol nasal irrigation in the management of chronic rhinosinusitis: a pilot study. Laryngoscope 2011; 121: 2468–2472

[16] Adappa ND, Wei CC, Palmer JN. Nasal irrigation with or without drugs: the evidence. Curr Opin Otolaryngol Head Neck Surg 2012; 20: 53–57

[17] Wei CC, Adappa ND, Cohen NA. Use of topical nasal therapies in the management of chronic rhinosinusitis. Laryngoscope 2013; 123: 2347–2359

[18] Campos J, Heppt W, Weber R. Nasal douches for diseases of the nose and the paranasal sinuses—a comparative in vitro investigation. Eur Arch Otorhinolaryngol 2013; 270: 2891–2899

[19] Zalmanovici Trestioreanu A, Yaphe J. Intranasal steroids for acute sinusitis. Cochrane Database Syst Rev 2013; 12: CD005149

[20] Mortuaire G, de Gabory L, François M et al. Rebound congestion and rhinitis medicamentosa: nasal decongestants in clinical practice. Critical review of the literature by a medical panel. Eur Ann Otorhinolaryngol Head Neck Dis 2013; 130: 137–144

[21] Autio-Gold J. The role of chlorhexidine in caries prevention. Oper Dent 2008; 33: 710–716

[22] Tuna A, Delilbasi C, Arslan A, Gurol Y, Tazegun Tekkanat Z. Do antibacterial mouthrinses affect bacteraemia in third molar surgery? A pilot study. Aust Dent J 2012; 57: 435–439

[23] Pilloni A, Zeza B, Mongardini C, Dominici F, Cassini MA, Polimeni A. A preliminary comparison of the effect of 0.3% versus 0.2% chlorhexidine mouth rinse on de novo plaque formation: a monocentre randomized double-blind crossover trial. Int J Dent Hyg 2013; 11: 198–202

[24] Casale M, Ciglia G, Frari V et al. The potential role of hyaluronic acid in postoperative radiofrequency surgery for chronic inferior turbinate hypertrophy. Am J Rhinol Allergy 2013; 27: 234–236

[25] Gelardi M, Guglielmi AV, De Candia N, Maffezzoni E, Berardi P, Quaranta N. Effect of sodium hyaluronate on mucociliary clearance after functional endoscopic sinus surgery. Eur Ann Allergy Clin Immunol 2013; 45: 103–108

[26] Grosjean P, Weber R. Fungus balls of the paranasal sinuses: a review. Eur Arch Otorhinolaryngol 2007; 264: 461–470 Review

[27] Ferreiro JA, Carlson BA, Cody DT III. Paranasal sinus fungus balls. Head Neck 1997; 19: 481–486

Chapter 6

Surgical Treatment

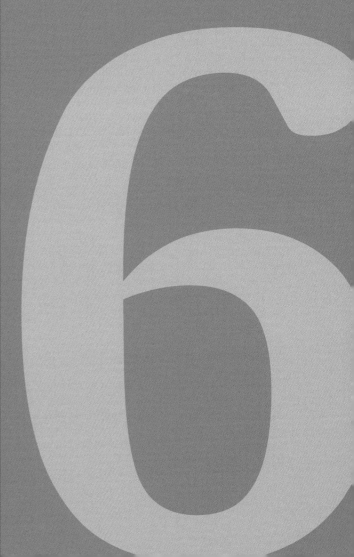

6 Surgical Treatment

Giovanni Felisati, Matteo Chiapasco, Federico Biglioli, Roberto Borloni, Paolo Lozza, Carlotta Pipolo, Marco Zaniboni

Contents Overview

In this section, the management of complications following: (1) "classic" odontogenic sinusitis; (2) infection of implants penetrating the maxillary sinus; and (3) infection of paranasal sinuses following migration/displacement of teeth/roots, implants, or materials used for sinus grafting procedures will be thoroughly analyzed.

Surgical Protocols According to Type of Complication

Surgical approaches vary considerably according to the etiological factors responsible for sinus infection (classical odontogenic infection, implants penetrating into the maxillary sinus, displaced/migrated implants or tooth/root fragments in the paranasal cavities, penetration into the maxillary sinus of materials used for sinus grafting procedures, presence or absence of involvement of other paranasal sinuses, presence or absence of oroantral communications).

Generally speaking, the first aim of treatment is to remove the main cause of infection. It is worth noting that in patients with infected or necrotic teeth responsible for an odontogenic sinusitis an attempt should always first be made to save the tooth (if not destroyed by significant decay and if a negotiable root canal system is present) with the correct endodontic treatment or re-treatment. In patients with damage to the periapical system, where it would be impossible or difficult to guarantee an adequate endodontic seal, apicoectomy of the involved roots is indicated. Neither endodontic treatment modalities nor apicoectomies will be described in detail, as a thorough explanation of these techniques is outside of the scope of this textbook.

Adequate antibiotic treatment should always be combined with the endodontic procedures to eliminate residual infection from the paranasal sinus system. For details, see Section 5.2.2 (p. 77) and Section 5.3.1 (p. 79). If endodontic treatment in association with antibiotic therapy does not lead to a remission of sinus infection, drainage of the residual infection can be performed via a transnasal endoscopic approach. For details, see Section 6.3 (p. 101) of this chapter.

When the tooth (or teeth) cannot be saved by endodontic treatment, the only way to resolve the sinusitis is by tooth extraction.

In patients with migrated or displaced implants, teeth, root fragments, endodontic materials, or grafting materials used for sinus floor elevation that have caused or may be followed by sinus infection, these foreign bodies should be removed as soon as possible.

The second objective is to guarantee adequate ventilation of the paranasal cavities and, finally, the third objective is to close oroantral communications (if any) created during tooth extraction or by incorrect surgical maneuvers during implant placement.

Three main surgical approaches are available: (1) intraoral surgical approaches; (2) transnasal endoscopic surgery; and (3) a combination of these two techniques. Every approach has specific indications, advantages, and limits: the aim of this chapter is to provide well-defined protocols, to enable the surgeon to choose the appropriate alternative according to the initial clinical situation (▶ Table 6.1 and ▶ Fig. 6.1).

6.1 Intraoral Approaches

6.1.1 Introduction

Intraoral approaches not associated with endoscopic sinus surgery are mainly indicated in the following clinical situations: (1) removal of infected teeth/roots still in their original position or displaced into the sinus and removal of endodontic materials displaced into the sinus; (2) removal of implants partially penetrating or completely displaced into the sinus and causing inflammatory or infectious reaction in the sinus that is not susceptible to medical treatment; (3) closure of oroantral communications with intraoral local flaps.

A prerequisite for the use of an intraoral approach only (not combined with transnasal endoscopic surgery) is the absence of severe sinusitis associated with obstruction of the maxillary ostium and/or involvement of other paranasal sinuses.

On the contrary, whenever the penetration/migration/displacement of infected teeth/roots or oral implants into the sinus is associated with significant sinus infection and obstruction of the ostium, or whenever other paranasal sinuses are involved, an intraoral approach alone may not be sufficient to re-establish normal function of the affected sinus (normal clearance and patency of the maxillary ostium) and does not allow treatment of infection involving other paranasal sinuses. In such patients, there is a potential risk of persistent infection, despite the removal of the foreign body. It is therefore mandatory to perform a thorough clinical and radiographic evaluation before deciding on the most appropriate approach. Traditional intraoral or panoramic radiographs are indicated to evaluate the condition of the teeth or implants and the surrounding alveolar bone, but are inadequate for evaluation of the sinonasal complex (▶ Fig. 6.2). For the latter, CT scans involving the whole sinonasal complex (including the cranial base) are fundamental in obtaining thorough and reliable information and thereby choosing the

Table 6.1 Surgical protocols according to type of complication

Group	Class	Condition	Treatment
1 – Complications following pre/peri-implant reconstructive procedures			
	1	Maxillary sinusitis following maxillary sinus lift (with or without involvement of other sinuses) with OAC	**Combined:** maxillary sinus FESS/extended FESS + infected material removal + OAC repair
2 – Complications following implant placement			
	2a	Peri-implantitis with sinusitis	**Combined:** FESS/extended FESS + removal of implant + OAC repair
	2b	Implant displacement with sinusitis and OAC	**Combined:** FESS/extended FESS + removal of implant + OAC repair
	2c	Implant displacement with maxillary sinusitis (with or without involvement of other sinuses)	**FESS:** endoscopic removal + maxillary sinus FESS/extended FESS
	2d	Implant displacement into the maxillary sinus or nasal cavity or other sinuses without sinusitis	Exclusive canine fossa approach with endoscopic aid or transnasal endoscopy with or without antrostomy depending on implant location
3 – "Classic" dental treatment complications			
	3a	Maxillary sinusitis (with or without involvement of other sinuses) (bacterial and/or fungal) with OAC	**Combined:** Maxillary sinus FESS/extended FESS (+ antibiotic therapy) + OAC repair + Treatment of the odontogenic focus
	3b	Maxillary sinusitis (with or without involvement of other sinuses) (bacterial and/or fungal)	Maxillary sinus FESS/extended FESS (+ antibiotic therapy) + Treatment of the odontogenic focus

Abbreviations: FESS, functional endoscopic sinus surgery; OAC, oroantral communication.

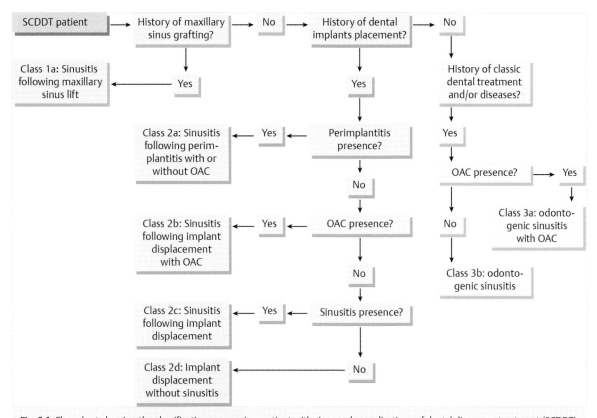

Fig. 6.1 Flow chart showing the classification process in a patient with sinonasal complications of dental disease or treatment (SCDDT).

most appropriate treatment modality (▶ Fig. 6.3). See Chapter 2 (p. 16) for more details.

Before proceeding with intraoral approaches, reduction of sinus infection (if any) is indicated, using adequate antibiotic therapy as described in Section 5.3.1 (p. 79).

See cases presented in ▶ Video 6.1, ▶ Video 6.2, ▶ Video 6.3, ▶ Video 6.4, ▶ Video 6.5, ▶ Video 6.6, ▶ Video 6.7, ▶ Video 6.8, ▶ Video 6.9, ▶ Video 6.10, ▶ Video 6.11, ▶ Video 6.12, ▶ Video 6.13, and ▶ Video 6.14.

6.1.2 Techniques

Removal of Infected Teeth/Roots Still in Their Original Position

As previously underlined, besides endodontic treatment of teeth that are infected but still have crowns and roots in good condition, extraction is the only treatment available for irreversibly compromised teeth or roots responsible for sinus infection (▶ Fig. 6.4).

Tooth/root extraction must be performed with levers and/or forceps according to routine extraction techniques. The only difference is that an oroantral communication may be created at the end of the procedure, because of the proximity of the root tips to the sinus floor. In such patients, the integrity or perforation of Schneider's membrane must be assessed, either by direct inspection or by Valsalva's maneuver.

If no oroantral communication is present after tooth/root extraction, no further procedures are indicated. Following extraction, the empty alveolar socket will be filled by a blood clot, which will progressively transform into granulation tissue and, finally, lead to new bone formation with socket closure.

If an oroantral communication is detected, two potential evolutions are possible: (1) spontaneous closure of the communication, due to organization of the blood clot in the alveolar socket and spontaneous

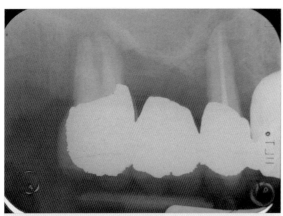

Fig. 6.2 Periapical radiograph showing periradicular radiolucency (sign of osteolysis) around 15 and 17, natural teeth supporting a fixed bridge, and opacity of the floor of the maxillary sinus. Due to the nature (2-dimensional image, intraoral positioning) and the limited dimensions of the image, it is impossible to properly evaluate the clinical situation.

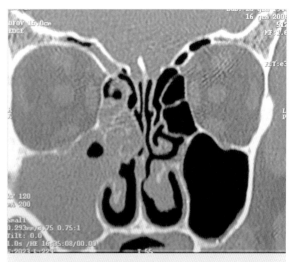

Fig. 6.3 CT scan of the same patient. The extension of the acquired volume allows an accurate examination of the clinical scenario: the radiopacity involves the entire lumen of the right maxillary sinus, together with several ethmoidal cells and the ipsilateral frontal sinus.

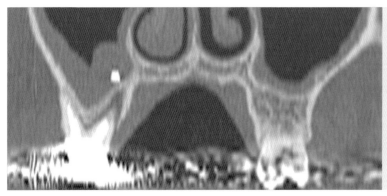

Fig. 6.4 CT scan showing complications following endodontic treatment: periradicular radiolucency (tooth 16) is visible, in association with a mass of radiopaque material dispersed inside the maxillary sinus and hypertrophy of the sinusal mucosa.

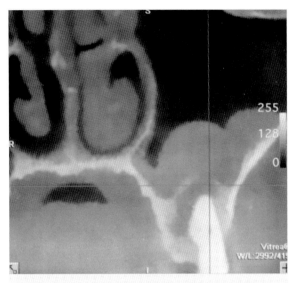

Fig. 6.5 CT scan showing periradicular radiolucency with interruption of the bony component of the sinusal floor and opacity at the bottom of the sinus.

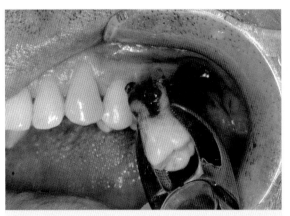

Fig. 6.6 The tooth is extracted with controlled movements, to avoid maneuvers that could enlarge the existing interruption of the sinusal floor.

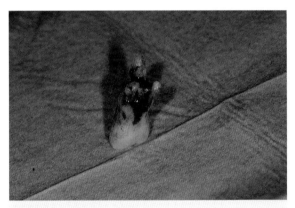

Fig. 6.7 The extracted tooth with a small portion of sinusal mucosa attached to one of the roots.

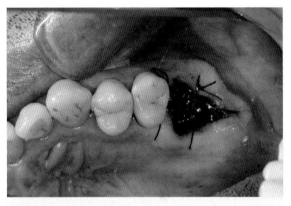

Fig. 6.8 This small oroantral communication will heal spontaneously through blood clotting and re-epithelialization. No additional surgical treatment is needed.

re-epithelialization over it (▶ Fig. 6.5, ▶ Fig. 6.6, ▶ Fig. 6.7, ▶ Fig. 6.8); and (2) persistence of the communication and transformation into an oroantral fistula.

The first scenario is more likely to occur in patients with small perforations, while the latter is frequently associated with larger communications. If not promptly treated, the communication may become irreversible, as a result of migration of the sinus epithelium and the oral mucosa into the communication, thus rendering a secondary spontaneous closure impossible, with the formation of an oroantral fistula (▶ Fig. 6.9, ▶ Fig. 6.10, ▶ Fig. 6.11). Whenever there is a high risk of this happening, closure of the oroantral communication should be performed immediately. Copious rinsing of the maxillary sinus cavity with sterile saline solution (with or without antibiotics) is recommended, in order to remove any infected

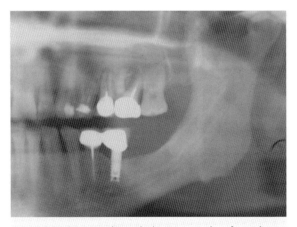

Fig. 6.9 Panoramic radiograph showing sequelae of complications following endodontic treatment of teeth 2.5 and 2.6. Both teeth must be extracted.

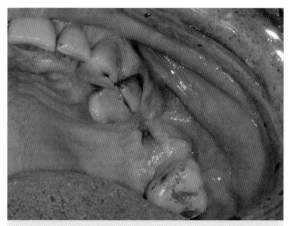

Fig. 6.10 Three weeks after the extraction a small oroantral communications has developed.

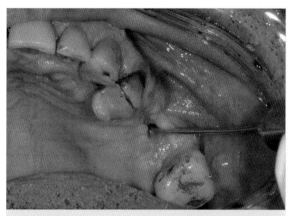

Fig. 6.11 The introduction of a blunt needle confirms the presence of the oroantral fistula.

material from the maxillary sinus and reduce the risk of relapse of sinusitis after surgery.

The closure of the communication is generally performed with local flaps. Among the different alternatives, a flap formed by local alveolar mucosa on the buccal side of the maxilla (the so-called Rehrmann flap) and the buccal fat pad flap are the most frequently used. The palatal flap and the lingual flap are less frequently used alternatives.

An oroantral communication may also develop as a consequence of either the removal of an implant penetrating into the sinus or the displacement/migration of teeth/roots or implants into the sinus. However, the techniques that can be used to close an oroantral communication will be described in detail in this section, with only brief reminders in the following sections.

Rehrmann flap

This flap is a full-thickness flap formed by the mucoperiosteum covering the buccal aspect of the maxillary bone. Briefly, an incision is made along the alveolar crest together with two vertical releasing incisions, approximately one centimeter distal and mesial to the oroantral communication, to guarantee reliable support to the flap at the end of surgery and adequate healing. A subperiosteal elevation is performed until the margins of the oroantral communication are identified, and every remnant of connective or soft tissue around and inside the communication is removed (▶ Fig. 6.12). The flap is released with periosteal incisions until a tension-free flap is obtained (▶ Fig. 6.13). To increase the possibility of a primary intention closure, a thin strip of mucosa is removed on the palatal side in such a way that the buccal flap may cover and overlap the oroantral communication. Mattress sutures are recommended, as they may reduce the risk of wound dehiscence during the early phases of

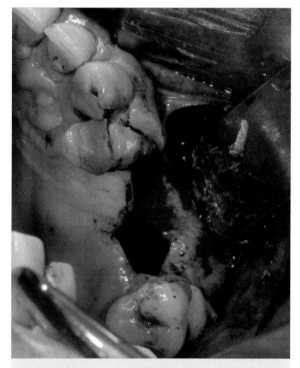

Fig. 6.12 After elevation of a full-thickness flap the exact extent of the oroantral communication is visible.

healing (▶ Fig. 6.14, ▶ Fig. 6.15). It is worth noting that root-form implants, once removed, leave only a circumferential and relatively small oroantral communication, which is quite easily closed. On the contrary, blade implants and in particular subperiosteal implants, which can become exposed in case of infection, may leave not only larger oroantral communications but also very irregular margins of the flaps and even a loss of soft tissues, which may render primary closure more difficult.

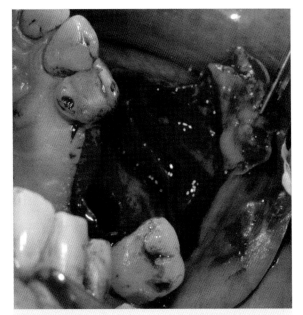

Fig. 6.13 After cautious curettage and irrigation with sterile saline inside the maxillary sinus, periosteal releasing incisions are performed on the buccal side of the surgical flap to allow the extension of the soft tissues over the oroantral communication.

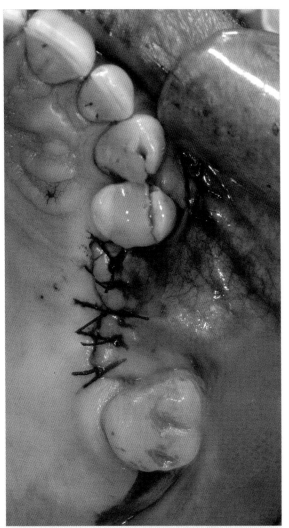

Fig. 6.14 Water-tight sutures are applied to prevent the passage of air and/or fluids from the mouth to the sinus and vice versa, which could compromise the healing process.

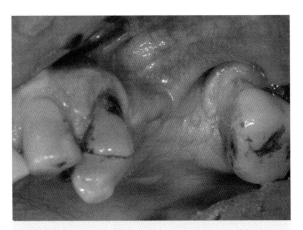

Fig. 6.15 One month after suture removal it is possible to confirm the complete healing of the soft tissues.

Buccal fat pad flap

The buccal fat pad, contained in a space delimited on its outer aspect by the masseter muscle, and on its inner aspect by the buccinator muscle, is an excellent source of well-vascularized tissue. It can be used alone, as it undergoes re-epithelialization on its surface quite rapidly, or in association with a Rehrmann flap.

The buccal fat pad is exposed through an incision of the periosteum in the buccal vestibule of the posterior maxilla and is easily identified immediately deep to this layer. The fat pad can then be isolated from the surrounding tissues with blunt dissection, taking care to maintain its vascular pedicle intact. This flap offers quite a considerable quantity of tissue that can easily be pulled and elongated to cover wide oroantral communications. Once its mobility has been checked, the flap can be sutured to the margins of the communication. As previously stated, this flap can be used alone or in association with the Rehrmann flap. In the latter case, the buccal fat pad forms the deeper layer, while the Rehrmann flap forms the outer layer. This combination is particularly indicated in patients with larger communications, where the risk of early wound dehiscence is higher, for instance in patients where removal of subperiosteal implants has caused chronic infection, implant exposure, and loss of soft tissues (► Fig. 6.16, ► Fig. 6.17, ► Fig. 6.18, ► Fig. 6.19).

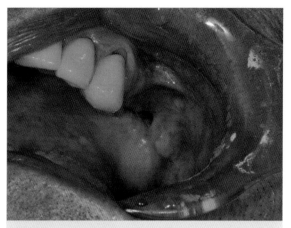

Fig. 6.16 Oroantral fistula following molar extraction.

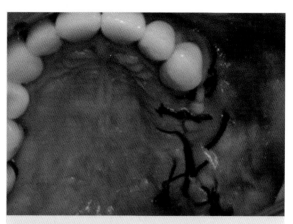

Fig. 6.18 The Rehrmann flap is sutured over the buccal fat pad flap.

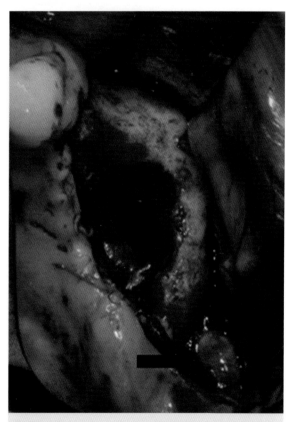

Fig. 6.17 The elevation of a full-thickness flap shows a wide bone defect. When bone loss is such that it can jeopardize the healing of the overlying soft tissues owing to insufficient support, the simultaneous use of two flaps may be indicated. The buccal fat pad (*arrow*) is identified and bluntly dissected in order to mobilize it until it allows the defect closure (deeper layer).

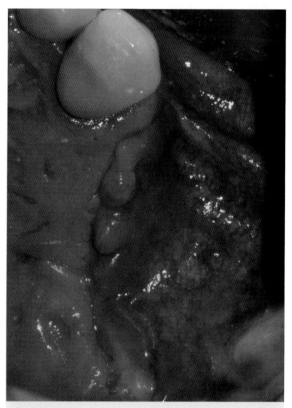

Fig. 6.19 Two weeks after suture removal the soft tissues have almost completely healed with disappearance of the oroantral fistula.

Palatal flap

This flap is a mucoperiosteal, full-thickness flap, supplied by the palatine artery. The flap is outlined with two parallel incisions, one along the alveolar crest of the maxilla and the second close to the palatal midline. The length of the flap varies according to surgical needs. A

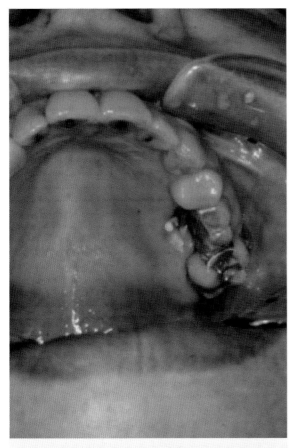

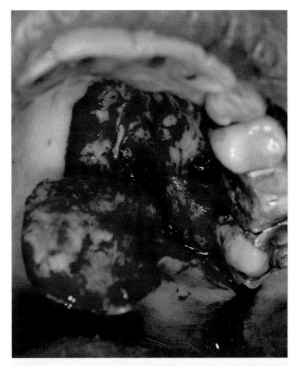

Fig. 6.21 After elevation of a full-thickness palatal flap the communication is exposed.

Fig. 6.20 Oroantral communication following root resection and extraction of the palatal root of 26.

subperiosteal dissection is performed, taking care to maintain the palatine artery intact and included in the flap (▶ Fig. 6.20, ▶ Fig. 6.21).

The flap is then rotated laterally until it covers the oroantral communication and sutured to the margins of the communication. The exposed palatal bone can be left to heal by secondary intention. Coverage of the exposed bone and re-epithelialization will occur spontaneously within a few weeks (▶ Fig. 6.22, ▶ Fig. 6.23, ▶ Fig. 6.24).

Although the quality of this flap is excellent, because of its thickness its mobility is limited, and therefore closure of oroantral communications, in particular if close to the base of the vascular pedicle, is not always easy to perform.

The palatal flap can also be combined with other local flaps, such as the Rehrmann or the buccal fat pad flap, but these procedures are seldom applied by oral and maxillofacial surgeons.

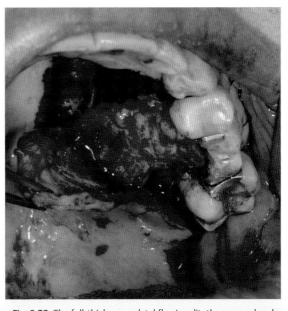

Fig. 6.22 The full-thickness palatal flap is split: the mucosal and submucosal layers are separated so that the latter can be moved more easily and can be sutured to the buccal side of the surgical flap to obtain coverage of the communication.

Lingual flap

The lingual flap is formed by a portion of the dorsal part of the tongue that remains pedicled to the tongue on one side and rotated toward the palate to close an oroantral communication. Nowadays this flap is very rarely used for the closure of oroantral communications, because of discomfort reported by patients in the weeks following

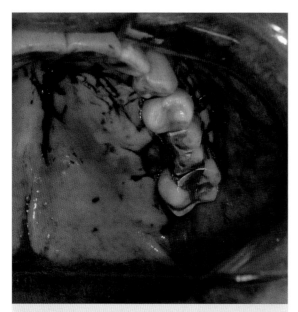

Fig. 6.23 The mucosal layer is repositioned with interdental sutures.

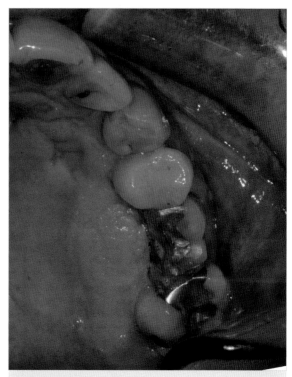

Fig. 6.24 Two months later the soft tissues have healed, completely obliterating the fistula.

surgery and the lack of any advantages compared with the previously described flaps.

Removal of Implants Penetrating into the Sinus and Causing Inflammatory/ Infectious Reaction in the Sinus

If an implant partially penetrates into the maxillary sinus and infection remains despite attempts to resolve it with medical therapy, the implant, although osseointegrated, should be removed as soon as possible. Surgical approaches differ according to the type of implant and its degree of stability. As previously stated, a thorough preoperative clinical and radiographic evaluation is fundamental. If CT scans show a completely opaque maxillary sinus, a nonpatent ostium, and eventual involvement of other paranasal sinuses, an intraoral approach alone is insufficient and must be combined with transnasal endoscopic surgery (FESS), in order to re-establish normal function and ventilation of the maxillary sinus, enlarge the natural ostium, and remove any infectious material from other paranasal sinuses not accessible from the oral cavity.

In a patient with a root-form implant, a first attempt can be made by unscrewing the implant. If the implant is no longer integrated or if the quantity of bone-to-implant contact is limited, this simple maneuver is effective in the majority of patients. Unscrewing an implant can be done with dental forceps or with dedicated instruments that can exert considerable torque on the implant, thereby facilitating its removal (▶ Fig. 6.25).

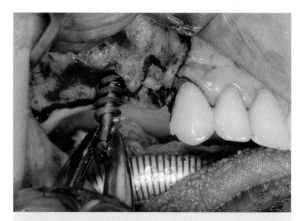

Fig. 6.25 An infected screw-type implant can be removed by unscrewing it with dental forceps if osseointegration is lost or bone-to-implant contact is reduced.

If this first maneuver fails, the suggested procedure is to remove a thin layer of bone around the implant: excessive use of forceps may lead to the fracture of the alveolar bone surrounding the implant and/or deformation and fracture of the implant, which may render complete removal of the implant difficult. This procedure can be accomplished with a variety of mechanical instruments, such as fissure burs or core drills assembled on dental handpieces (▸ Fig. 6.26, ▸ Fig. 6.27), or with piezoelectric instruments.

It is strongly recommended that a full-thickness local flap is raised to control the surgical field and to prepare favorable conditions for the following phase, namely closure of the oroantral communication that inevitably develops following implant removal.

The removal of peri-implant bone will weaken the bone-to-implant contact and simplify removal of the implant. Whatever instrument is used, this procedure must be performed under constant irrigation with sterile, cold saline solution, to avoid overheating of the surrounding bone. Nowadays, piezoelectric instruments are likely to guarantee a less aggressive approach with preservation of more alveolar bone. It is worth noting that some of these patients may be potential candidates for a new implant placement procedure. If significant loss of the alveolar bone has been caused by improper maneuvers, the residual bone may be insufficient to host new implants, unless more complex reconstructive procedures are performed.

Other types of implants such as blade or subperiosteal implants cannot be removed with unscrewing maneuvers because of their shape. Blade and subperiosteal implants, which are often not osseointegrated, but generally surrounded by thick connective tissue, must be separated by dissection with elevators or scissors from this tissue, which tends to incorporate the implants and render their removal more difficult and time-consuming (▸ Fig. 6.28, ▸ Fig. 6.29, ▸ Fig. 6.30). These implants tend to cause greater peri-implant bone resorption/destruction once they become infected, thus creating wider oroantral communications compared with root-form implants.

Once the implant has been removed, a careful curettage must be performed to remove any residual infected connective or soft tissues surrounding the implant site (▸ Fig. 6.31). As an unavoidable consequence of implant removal, an oroantral communication will occur in most patients. Irrigation of the sinus and suctioning through the oroantral communication is recommended, in order to remove any infected material from the maxillary sinus. Finally, the oroantral communication must be hermetically closed with a local flap, as already described in the previous section (▸ Fig. 6.32, ▸ Fig. 6.33).

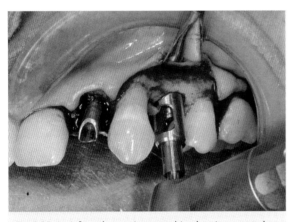

Fig. 6.26 An infected, osseointegrated implant is separated from the surrounding bone with the use of a core drill. The diameter of the drill is chosen according to the diameter of the implant, to avoid any unnecessary bone loss.

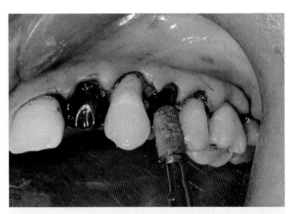

Fig. 6.27 After circumferential osteotomy with the core drill the implant can be unscrewed with an appropriate ratchet wrench.

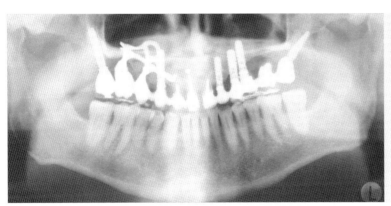

Fig. 6.28 Panoramic radiograph showing the penetration of a subperiosteal implant into the lumen of the right maxillary sinus.

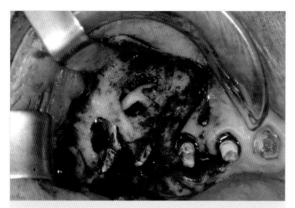

Fig. 6.29 After elevation of a full-thickness flap it is possible to evaluate the extent of the bone loss and the oroantral communications.

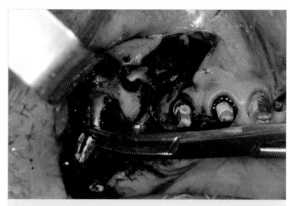

Fig. 6.30 The subperiosteal implant must be separated into pieces with an appropriate bur mounted on surgical straight handpieces to be extracted from the maxillary sinus.

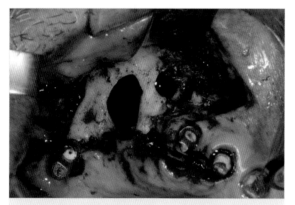

Fig. 6.31 After removal of the infected implant, the sinus is irrigated with sterile saline and a careful curettage of the bony communications is performed.

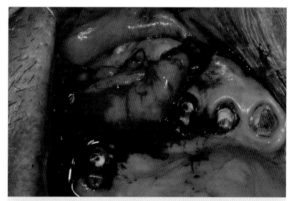

Fig. 6.32 Owing to the extent of the oroantral communication, the retrieval and use of the buccal fat pad is mandatory. The fat pad acts as a support layer for the overlying mucosa.

Removal of Teeth/Roots, Endodontic Materials, or Implants Displaced/Migrated into the Maxillary Sinus

As described in detail in Chapter 3 (p. 40), displacement of teeth/roots, endodontic materials, or implants into the maxillary sinus may be followed by: (1) spontaneous expulsion through the antrum; (2) persistence of these foreign bodies in the sinus without infection; or (3) a foreign body reaction with infection that may involve the maxillary sinus only, other paranasal sinuses, the orbit, and finally, the endocranial content. The second and third scenarios may be followed by major complications such as orbital cellulitis, optic nerve infection, and potentially life-threatening intracranial infections. In order to avoid these serious complications, it is recommended that foreign bodies are removed from the maxillary sinus as soon as possible.

As previously stated, an intraoral approach is indicated whenever the presence of foreign bodies in the maxillary sinus is not associated with severe sinusitis, obstruction of the ostium, or involvement of other paranasal sinuses.

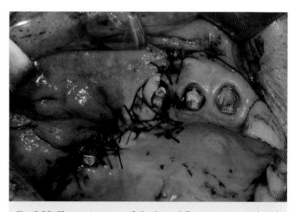

Fig. 6.33 The periosteum of the buccal flap is interrupted and the flap is extended over the fat pad layer, to be sutured to the palatal mucosa.

Different techniques have been proposed over the years, including: (1) immediate removal of a tooth/root or implant through the oroantral communication created by incorrect maneuvers during implant placement or tooth extraction; (2) an intraoral Caldwell–Luc operation[2–4] with removal of part of the anterior-lateral wall of the maxillary sinus; (3) an intraoral approach with the creation of a bony window pedicled to Schneider's membrane[5,6]; and, finally, (4) Caldwell–Luc operation with endoscopic removal via an intraoral approach through the anterior wall of the maxillary sinus.[7,8]

Immediate removal of a tooth/root or implant through the oroantral communication created by incorrect maneuvers during implant placement or tooth extraction

As a consequence of bad planning and improper surgical maneuvers, an implant or a tooth can be displaced into the sinus. Through the oroantral communication that will be inevitably created, an attempt can be made to remove the displaced foreign body before adopting more invasive procedures.

If this maneuver is performed immediately after the complication occurs, there is a chance that the foreign body is still close to the floor of the maxillary sinus. Using a curved curette or by irrigation with saline solution and suctioning with a high-speed suctioning tip (or using both techniques) it may be possible to remove the foreign body before it migrates to a different position as a result of the patient's movements and/or ciliary activity, which tend to cause the foreign body to migrate toward the maxillary ostium.

If this maneuver is successful, after removal of the foreign body and irrigation with sterile saline, the oroantral communication can be closed with a local flap as previously described. However, the likelihood of successful treatment is relatively low, because the narrowness of the access limits visibility and maneuverability during retrieval of the foreign body. Moreover, the foreign body may quickly migrate into areas of the sinus that are inaccessible. Endoscopy performed through the oroantral communication can improve the technique and maximize the chances of removing the foreign body; however, immediate maneuvers to address these clinical problems are generally the responsibility of dentists who have no optical endoscopes in their cabinets and no experience of endoscopy. In future it may be desirable for every dental practice to have a 4-mm, 0° optical endoscope for this purpose. This maneuver can be performed under local anesthesia.

Intraoral Approach using a Caldwell–Luc Operation

The Caldwell–Luc operation, which uses an intraoral approach with removal of part of the anterolateral wall of the maxillary sinus and part of the sinus mucosa[2–4] is the second available alternative for removing displaced or migrated teeth/roots and implants.

Immediately prior to the surgical procedure, a panoramic radiograph is generally performed, to verify the position of the foreign body in the maxillary sinus. It is well known that mucociliary activity of the sinus mucosa and patient movements may cause significant changes in the position of the foreign body within hours or days and may even lead to extrusion of the foreign body from the sinus. According to the information provided by this radiograph, the area of bone removal from the anterolateral wall of the maxillary sinus that is necessary to access the sinus can vary significantly.

The majority of patients can be treated with local anesthesia. Sedation or general anesthesia is only indicated for noncompliant patients. Local anesthesia is achieved with injection of local anesthetic in association with epinephrine (to obtain vasoconstriction and better hemostasis) in the buccal sulcus of the anterolateral maxilla. If necessary, this anesthesia can be associated with a block of the main trunk of the infraorbital nerve, responsible for the innervation of the alveolar/maxillary bone, the surrounding soft tissues, and Schneider's membrane. Anesthesia can be obtained through an intraoral approach or directly around and inside the infraorbital foramen via a percutaneous approach.

Access to the anterolateral wall of the maxillary sinus is obtained in different ways, mainly depending on the presence or absence of an oroantral communication or fistula. In fact, the diagnosis of displacement of teeth/roots or implants into the maxillary sinus may be made when it first occurs, but also at a later stage. In the latter situation, the presence of the foreign body in the sinus may not be associated with an oroantral communication, owing to spontaneous closure or sometimes immediate closure performed by the dentist. In addition, displacement of endodontic material into the sinus, due to incorrect or excessive filling of the root canal system following disruption of the periapical seal, develops without any oroantral communication.

In the presence of an oroantral communication, the incision line must follow the margins of the communication or fistula (generally, but not always, on the midline of the alveolar crest) and it then continues mesial and distal to the communication. Vertical releasing incisions are performed in order to gain access to the anterolateral wall of the maxillary sinus. If a true fistula (characterized by epithelialization of the communication) is present, this tissue must be carefully removed. If no oroantral communication or fistula is present, a midcrestal incision and vertical releasing incisions are performed. In order to guarantee better healing, it is strongly suggested that the vertical incisions are outlined at least one centimeter mesial and distal to the expected location of the bony window necessary to access the sinus.

A mucoperiosteal flap is then raised and the maxillary bone exposed. The elevation is generally extended upward until the infraorbital nerve is identified. The flap is retracted, maintaining two retractors medial and distal to the nerve, to avoid any compression or traction on it.

A bony window is outlined and part of the anterolateral wall of the maxillary sinus removed: the position and dimensions of this window will vary according to the foreign body position and surgical needs.

Schneider's membrane is sharply dissected in order to access the sinus. In this way, an excellent view of the maxillary sinus is obtained and the foreign body can be identified and removed. It is worth noting that, in contrast to the original approach described by Caldwell and Luc, there is no need to remove the mucosa of the rest of the sinus, even if it is thickened or has a polypoid appearance because of an inflammatory reaction. If the ostium is patent and once the foreign body is removed, spontaneous regression of these signs is likely to occur. Similarly, it is unnecessary, and indeed absolutely contraindicated, to perform the classic opening between the sinus and the nose used by otolaryngologists in the inferior meatus before the advent of the endoscope.

After inspection of the sinus and irrigation with sterile saline and/or antibiotic solutions, the flap is replaced in its original position and sutured, in order to guarantee a watertight closure. Periosteal releasing incisions are mandatory.

Compared with the approach through the oroantral communication, this approach allows excellent access and visual control of the maxillary sinus, rendering the removal of foreign bodies displaced into the sinus very easy (▶ Fig. 6.34, ▶ Fig. 6.35, ▶ Fig. 6.36, ▶ Fig. 6.37, ▶ Fig. 6.38).

However, this approach will leave a bone defect in the anterolateral wall of the maxillary sinus, which may lead to the formation of scar tissue, and later to the retraction of the soft tissues of the cheek and to paresthesia and pain if the infraorbital nerve branches are involved.[9–12] Moreover, the removal of sinus mucosa and the formation of scar tissue may render a sinus lift procedure difficult (if indicated in a second stage), even a long time after the

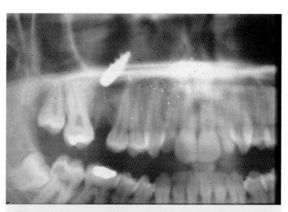

Fig. 6.34 Displacement of an implant into the maxillary sinus.

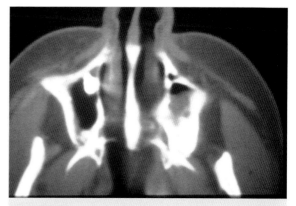

Fig. 6.35 CT scan showing the position of the implant and the lack of an inflammatory reaction inside the sinus.

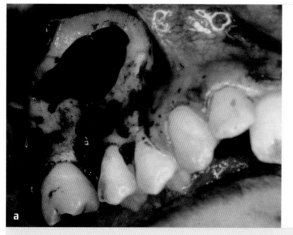

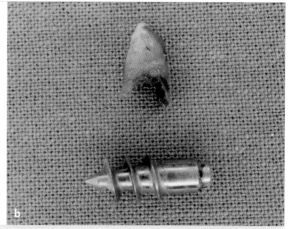

Fig. 6.36 (a,b) Removal of the implant through a Caldwell–Luc antrostomy procedure and extraction of an infected root.

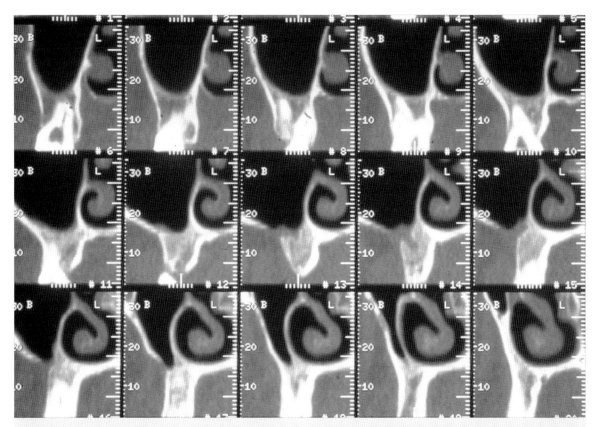

Fig. 6.37 CT scan 6 months later showing a completely aerated and healthy maxillary sinus.

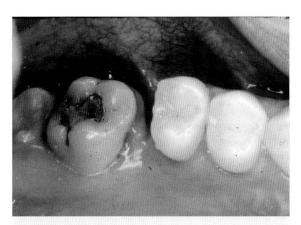

Fig. 6.38 Clinical control 6 months later showing complete closure of oroantral communication.

removal of an implant from the sinus. Consequently, alternative techniques have been proposed to avoid these complications.

Some authors have proposed replacing the lost antero-lateral sinus wall by means of a titanium mesh.[13] Unfortunately, this had to be removed in more than 50% of patients following infection and painful scarring reactions.[14]

Other authors[15,16] proposed completely removing the bony window to approach the maxillary sinus and replacing it after removal of the foreign body. The bony window was rigidly stabilized with metal wires. However, the main drawback was the high rate of sequestration of the bony window followed by infection, due to the scarce or absent revascularization of the bone lid.[17]

Intraoral approach with creation of a bony window pedicled to Schneider's membrane

This technique has been proposed to avoid the aforementioned disadvantages of the Caldwell–Luc operation, and consists of the creation of a bony window pedicled and vascularized by Schneider's membrane.[5,6]

As in the Caldwell–Luc technique, the majority of patients can be treated under local anesthesia, and the same procedure is used for injection of local anesthetic. In addition, the intraoral access to the anterolateral wall of the maxillary sinus and the elevation and retraction of the mucoperiosteal flap are similar to those described in the previous section for this technique.

A surgical felt-tip pen can be used over the anterolateral sinus wall to draw a rectangle of at least 2.5 × 1.5 cm in size. Its position and extent vary according to the

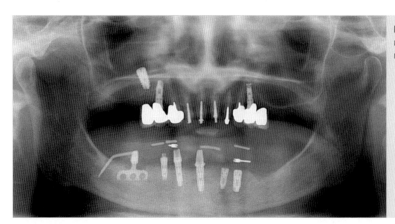

Fig. 6.39 Panoramic radiograph showing a root-form implant inside the lumen of the right maxillary sinus.

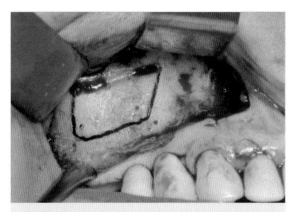

Fig. 6.40 On the lateral wall of the maxillary sinus, three complete and one (upper) incomplete osteotomy lines define a bony lid. Two small holes are created at the lower corners of the bony lid, coupled with two similar holes in the nearby area of the maxillary bone, to be used for lid repositioning.

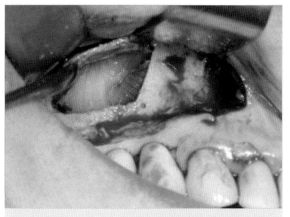

Fig. 6.41 The bone lid, pedicled to Schneider's membrane on the upper side, is pulled open to gain access to the lumen of the maxillary sinus and visualize the migrated implant.

dimensions of the sinus and the position of the foreign body. The first step of the procedure consists of the creation of two pairs of holes with a small diameter round bur, two of them just above and two just below the inferior margin of the rectangle. This maneuver is performed to allow the stabilization of the bony window with sutures at the end of the surgical procedure, but must be performed at the start, when the bone is stable.

The second step consists of the creation of osteotomy lines following the previously designed rectangle. The vertical (mesial and distal) and lower horizontal osteotomies can be performed with fine-diameter reciprocating saws or with piezoelectric instruments under constant irrigation with sterile saline and include both the bony wall of the maxillary sinus and the underlying Schneider's membrane, taking care to cut the membrane but not tear it. Conversely, the upper horizontal osteotomy of the bony window can be performed with a diamond bur assembled on a straight handpiece (or with piezoelectric instruments) in order to cut the bone but leave the sinus mucosa intact. This maneuver closely

resembles the preparation of the bony window used for a typical sinus lift procedure and the aims are: (1) to maintain a mucosal hinge, allowing mobilization of the bony window with an upward and inward or outward rotation; and (2) to ensure the vascularity of the bony window, thereby avoiding postoperative resorption or sequestration of the bony window (▶ Fig. 6.39, ▶ Fig. 6.40).

Once the window is rotated either inward or outward, the sinus cavity can be viewed directly. The foreign body can then be identified and removed either with a suctioning tip or surgical pliers (▶ Fig. 6.41, ▶ Fig. 6.42).

If the foreign body is surrounded by a reactive hypertrophic/hyperplastic sinus mucosa, this may be removed with delicate curettage, but no attempt to remove the whole sinus mucosa is indicated. Very frequently, this reactive thickening of the sinus mucosa will regress spontaneously once the foreign body has been removed, as demonstrated by CT scans performed at a later date.

Abundant rinsing of the maxillary sinus cavity is then performed with sterile saline solution (with or without antibiotics) to reduce the preexisting and potential bacterial contamination of the sinus cavity.

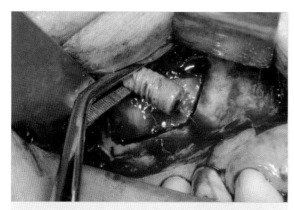

Fig. 6.42 The implant, thanks to the wide access to the sinusal lumen, is easily retrieved with a pair of pliers.

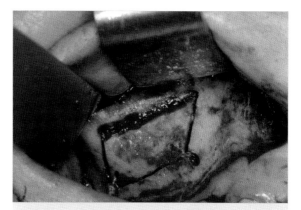

Fig. 6.43 The bone lid is repositioned and held in place with resorbable sutures engaging the small holes created in the lower corners of the lid and in nearby points of the maxillary bone.

Resorbable sutures are passed through the previously created holes to reposition the bony window in its original location: stabilization is guaranteed by the mucosal hinge superiorly and through tightening of the sutures inferiorly (▶ Fig. 6.43). Finally, the procedure is completed by suturing of the mucoperiosteal flap (▶ Fig. 6.44).

The advantages of this procedure can be summarized as follows: (1) the subperiosteal dissection limits bleeding and optimizes access to the anterolateral wall of the maxillary sinus; (2) the vascularization provided by the sinus mucosa ensures the survival of the bony window (with no significant resorption) and allows ossification of the margins of the bony window; (3) the procedure can be performed under local anesthesia in a relatively short operating time (20–30 minutes), with reduction of postoperative morbidity (particularly swelling); (4) the rapid healing of the sinus mucosa and the frequently complete reossification of the bony lid margins may allow, if indicated, a safe sinus lift procedure via a lateral approach, as in a previously untreated maxillary sinus.

Endoscopic removal via an intraoral approach through the anterior wall of the maxillary sinus

Described by Stammberger as a part of functional endoscopic sinus surgery,[18] this approach can be performed under local anesthesia with or without sedation in adults and/or combined with a block of the extraorbital trunk of the infraorbital nerve, as previously described. However, this procedure can also be used to remove implants,[8,19] in addition to any other foreign body, such as teeth, roots, or sinus grafting materials, displaced or migrated into the maxillary sinus.

This transoral canine fossa endoscopic approach was classically proposed with the use of a standard trocar and its sleeve, which penetrated the anterior wall of the maxillary sinus. However, this setup is limiting when attempting to perform more advanced surgical

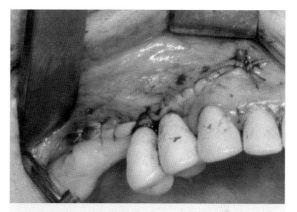

Fig. 6.44 The surgical flap is sutured.

procedures inside the sinus.[18] To overcome these limitations (loss of visualization during insertion of instruments and the narrow port), our group introduced the antral retriever, a specially designed trocar and sleeve.[7] The distal part of the sleeve of this device has a funnel shape to allow easy movement of any instrument. The proximal part, which crosses the bone when positioned, holds a lateral window. When the sheath is placed in the canine fossa, the sinus can be visualized using an endoscope and the simultaneously inserted operating instruments can easily move inside the maxillary sinus through the opening of the lateral window of the sleeve. The trocar has a diameter of 5 mm, and therefore a 4-mm endoscope (0° or angled) can be used for sinus surgery. Smaller endoscopes (e.g., 3 mm) and different angulation of the endoscope lens permit even better movement of the instruments under visualization. The insertion technique is the same as for traditional trocars.

This procedure can easily be performed under local anesthesia in the majority of patients. Anesthesia is obtained with local injection in the area to be treated

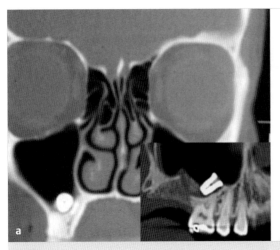
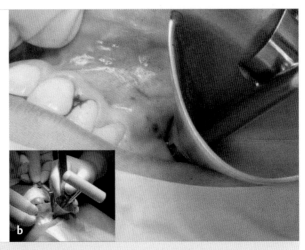

Fig. 6.45 **(a)** A case of canine fossa approach: CT scan of implant displaced into the right maxillary sinus during a mini sinus lift procedure with immediate loading. No maxillary sinusitis is present. **(b)** Antral retriever with trocar in place, positioned in the canine fossa.

either alone or combined with a block of the extraorbital trunk of the infraorbital nerve, as previously described.

In the absence of an oroantral communication, access to the anterior wall is obtained through a small incision in the buccal sulcus in the region of the canine fossa. In a patient with an oroantral communication, a full-thickness flap is raised as previously described for the other intraoral approaches, in order to close the communication at the end of surgery.

The antral retriever is then inserted into the oroantral communication or, in its absence, pushed into the maxillary sinus using cautious rotatory movements. After positioning, the endoscope (0–45° scope; 3–4 mm) is used to visualize the foreign bodies and Blakesley forceps (straight or upturned), or an equivalent instrument, are used to extract them under direct endoscopic visualization. Sinus lavage with saline through the retriever is also possible. Finally, the antral retriever is retracted and the access sutured (▶ Fig. 6.45, ▶ Fig. 6.46). This approach also allows the removal of alloplastic materials inserted together with the migrated implant during a transalveolar elevation of maxillary sinus, as described in Chapter 3 (p. 40).

The advantages of this technique are that good visualization of the sinus is achieved through a small surgical access and postoperative recovery is favorable, with limited pain and swelling. However, the control of the surgical field may be limited and foreign bodies displaced into the posterior and/or upper part of the maxillary sinus may not be easily reached. Therefore, in our hands, the indication to perform an endoscopic canine fossa approach (using the antral retriever) to remove migrated implants is limited to patients without any kind of sinusitis and, if present, only a small amount of migrated allogeneic material without alteration of the sinus floor structure.

6.1.3 Clinical Cases (History, Imaging, Treatment, Outcome)

Intraoral Approach: Case 1

The patient, a 61-year-old woman, had received, several years previously, six screw-type implants supporting a fixed complete prosthetic rehabilitation in the upper maxilla. After several episodes of local infection around the implant in position 16, the patient reported hearing a sharp noise while chewing soft food and, in the evening, the feeling of something rolling inside the maxilla when she lay down in bed. The patient decided to seek a specialist's advice and came to our attention. The case is shown in ▶ Fig. 6.47 a–i.

Intraoral Approach: Case 2

The patient, a 49-year-old man, was referred by a dentist for treatment of an odontogenic infection involving the roots of the upper left premolars and molars (25, 26, 27, 28) and the surrounding bone. The case is shown in ▶ Fig. 6.48 a–m.

Key Points

- How to manage oroantral communications following removal of implants, roots, and teeth via an intraoral approach.
- How to manage foreign bodies displaced/migrated into the maxillary sinus via an intraoral approach (with or without endoscopy).
- Advantages and disadvantages of intraoral approaches.

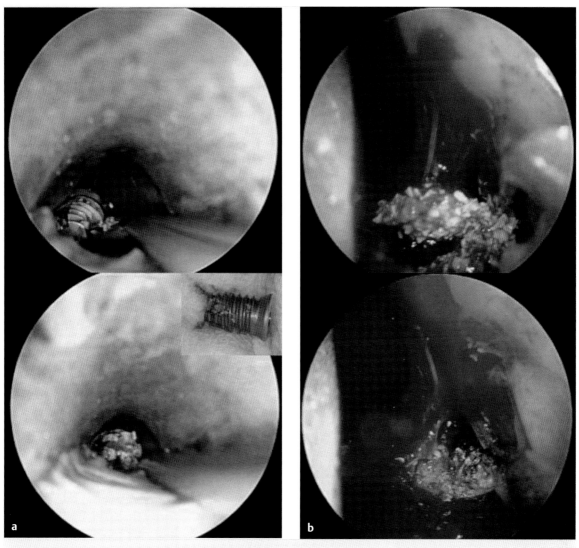

Fig. 6.46 (a) Endoscopic view after positioning of the antral retriever. Simultaneous grasping of the migrated implant and endoscopic visualization through the antral retriever. **(b)** Removal of the lifting material under visualization.

6.2 Transnasal Endoscopic Surgery

6.2.1 Introduction

Functional endoscopic sinus surgery (FESS) is still a relatively recent advancement in the treatment of a variety of sinonasal pathologies. Pioneered by Messerklinger in the late 1960s and spread throughout the surgical world by Stammberger[18] and Kennedy, this technique is based on an understanding of the mucociliary clearance pattern of sinuses toward their natural ostia, irrespective of additional openings. This knowledge, together with the constant innovation of instrumentation dedicated to endoscopic surgery, has made FESS and/or endoscopic sinus surgery (ESS) the gold standard for the treatment of

chronic sinusitis. Furthermore, as our knowledge of paranasal sinus anatomy has improved, other ancillary surgeries have developed, including endoscopic lacrimal surgery, orbital decompression, applications to the pterygopalatine and infratemporal fossae, and approaches from the sphenoid/sella extending to the cribriform, parasellar, and clival regions.

ESS has also gained a solid reputation in the treatment of extended disease of the sinuses as a consequence of the continuous implementation of new tools, devices, and techniques. Foremost, the advent of multi-angled endoscopes that provide excellent visualization of the nasal cavities, recesses of the maxillary sinus (alveolar recesses), and the frontal sinus allows the surgeon to reach these previously endoscopically hidden areas using dedicated curved instruments. This has enabled

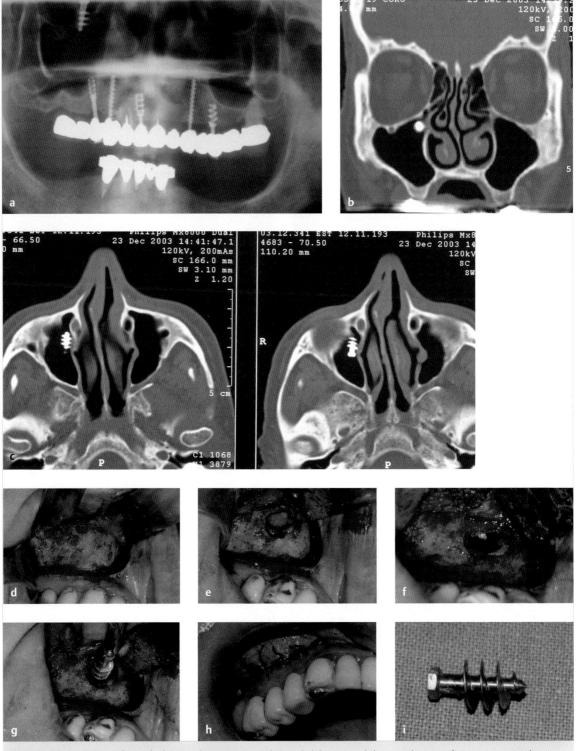

Fig. 6.47 (a) Panoramic radiograph showing the existent prosthetic rehabilitation and the partial image of a screw-type implant displaced into the upper third of the maxillary sinus. **(b,c)** Coronal and axial CT scans showing the exact position of the migrated implant near the natural ostium of the maxillary sinus. **(d,e)** A full-thickness mucoperiosteal flap is elevated and the lateral wall of the sinus is exposed. With the use of surgical burs mounted on a straight handpiece, an adequate osteotomy is performed to allow the identification and retrieval of the implant. **(f,g)** The displaced implant is located and extracted from the maxillary sinus with a pair of curved surgical pliers. **(h)** The surgical access is closed with interrupted silk sutures. **(i)** The retrieved implant.

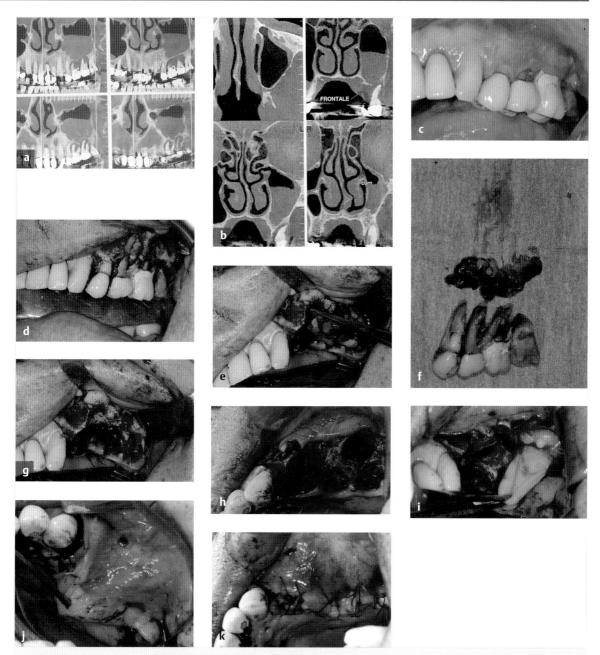

Fig. 6.48 **(a,b)** CT scans showing the loss of alveolar bone around the roots of 25, 26, 27, and 28, interruption of the bony floor of the maxillary sinus around 27, and a radiopacity involving the lower two-thirds of the sinusal lumen. **(c)** Intraoral view of the involved teeth: it is possible to note the recession of the soft tissues around the roots and the abundant calculus deposits. **(d)** After the elevation of a full-thickness flap the extent of the buccal alveolar bone loss and root exposure are clearly visible. **(e,f)** All the involved teeth are extracted and the granulation tissue surrounding the roots is enucleated. **(g,h)** After the complete removal of the infected tissues, thorough curettage of the residual bone and irrigation with sterile saline, the loss of alveolar bone and the extent of the oroantral communication are evaluated. **(i–k)** The buccal fat pad is partially extracted from its location to be used as a supporting layer for the overlying mucosa. The fat pad is sutured to the palatal mucosa and, on the buccal side of the surgical flap, the periosteal layer is interrupted to obtain an extension of the mucosa, thus allowing a tension-free suture of the Rehrmann flap over the fat pad layer.

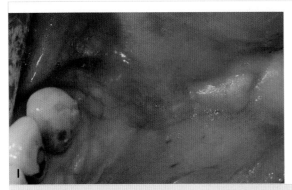
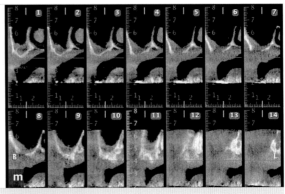

Fig. 6.48 (*Continued*) (**l,m**) One month after suture removal, complete healing of the treated area is assessed both clinically and radiographically.

endoscopic surgeons to focus on direct approaches through the natural ostia, even for these formerly inaccessible areas, and avoid in the majority of patients approaches such as the Caldwell–Luc procedure,[20] inferior meatal antrostomies, canine fossa punctures/approaches[21] (for the maxillary sinus), and external approaches to the frontal sinus.

The main advantages of FESS versus the classical open approaches to the maxillary sinus are the reduced invasiveness, the preservation of sinus anatomy and physiology, and the reduction in recovery times. Of utmost importance, however, when considering the matter at hand, is also the chance to speed up the prosthetic oral rehabilitation of the patient.[22]

This section will focus on transnasal endoscopic approaches to the maxillary sinus and will describe the basic techniques to improve ventilation of the ethmoid, sphenoid, and frontal sinuses. Furthermore, we will take into account the distinct endoscopic approaches required for treating SCDDT in accordance with the proposed classification.

6.2.2 Surgical Techniques

In the following paragraphs, a step-by-step approach to endoscopic sinus surgery procedures will be described in detail, starting with the preparation of the patient and basic FESS.

Presurgical Planning and Preparation

As underlined in previous chapters, thorough preoperative evaluation by endoscopy and imaging (CT/MRI) is mandatory. For example, the extent of inflammatory involvement of paranasal sinuses or the exact position of migrated materials must be assessed both via CT and nasal endoscopy, in order to efficiently plan the procedure and foresee possible complications and difficulties.

Furthermore, the outcome of preoperative evaluation also affects the choice of anesthesia for transnasal endoscopic approaches. In the early years of FESS, surgery was typically performed under local anesthesia with sedation; this was possible as the approaches were quite limited both in nature and in surgical time required. In recent years, however, the expansion of surgical possibilities and the introduction of total intravenous anesthesia (TIVA) with the associated reduction in blood loss[23] have led to a shift toward general anesthesia. However, in the specific field of migrated or displaced teeth/roots, endodontic materials, or dental implants, the choice of local or general anesthesia is determined by the position of the foreign body: materials displaced into or near the nasal cavity can usually be removed under local anesthesia with or without sedation.

Another crucial area is the medical treatment and preparation of the patient, including antibiotic and glucocorticoid therapy from 1 week prior to the surgery, as described in Chapter 5 (p. 76), to diminish the blood flow resulting from inflammation of the mucosa and reduce intraoperative bleeding, enhancing visibility in the operative field.

Finally, intranasal vasoconstriction before and during surgery is essential for a safe and efficacious outcome. This is best achieved by the intranasal placement of patties impregnated with topical solutions such as Xylocaine 5% with naphazoline. The application should be performed slowly and always while monitoring the patient for any change in blood pressure and heart rate.

Uncinectomy

Uncinectomy is considered the first step in the approach to the natural ostium of the maxillary sinus. Depending on the extent of the disease, a partial uncinectomy (the middle and horizontal part) may be sufficient to expose the ostium and induce correct ventilation and drainage of the sinus.

First, using a 0° endoscope, the position of the uncinate process should be assessed and, when in doubt, palpated with a ball-tipped right-angled probe. After identification, removal can be achieved either via an anterior approach, with incision using a sickle knife posterior to the frontal process of the maxilla and resection of the uncinate process from its superior and inferior portion, or through a retrograde removal of the free edge of the process. After medialization of the middle turbinate (▶ Fig. 6.49) a back-biting instrument is placed into the semilunar hiatus at the height of the floor of the ethmoidal bulla, engaging and removing the uncinate process backward as far as the frontal process of the maxilla (▶ Fig. 6.50 a–d). For the last bite, the backbiter should be moved upward toward the cranial part of the uncinate process to protect the nasolacrimal duct from injury. Next, fracture at its lateral and inferior attachment through an anterior movement of the engaged backbiter, curette, or ball probe exposes the residual medial and horizontal part of the process. The medial part is then removed with a 45°-angled through-cutting instrument and the horizontal part with the microdebrider, taking care to engage only the mobile part of the uncinate process, to avoid penetration into the lamina papyracea.

Behind the horizontal portion of the uncinate process lies the natural ostium, which at this point will still have untouched mucosal borders. Pivotal to the recognition of the natural ostium is its tilted angle, which distinguishes it from accessory ostia that, conversely, lie on a completely sagittal plane (▶ Fig. 6.51).

The danger points of this procedure are the nasolacrimal duct anteriorly and the lamina papyracea and orbit medially.

Antrostomy

The extent of a well-performed and effective antrostomy is still a matter of discussion. Some research groups focus on the lowering of nitric oxide (NO) concentrations and subsequent potential alteration in local innate defense should the antrostomy be too large,[24] while others focus on alteration of airflow into the maxillary sinus after antrostomy. Current consensus, however, states that the size of the opening should be dependent on the degree of the disease.[25,26]

Nevertheless, in our specific field, ventilation of the maxillary sinus is not the only objective to be achieved: often removal of foreign bodies is the main aim of the procedure. Therefore, the size of the antrostomy is highly dependent on the maneuverability of curved instruments in the alveolar recess: widening of the antrostomy often becomes necessary to reach the less accessible parts.

Identification of the correct location of the natural ostium is mandatory (▶ Fig. 6.52), as enlargement of an accessory ostium or creation of an artificial ostium without connection to the natural opening may result in failure of the procedure due to recirculation of the sinus content between the two ostia.

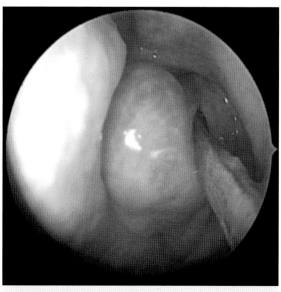

Fig. 6.49 Delicate medialization with a Freer elevator of the left middle turbinate to access the middle meatus.

When necessary, widening of the natural ostium is achieved after uncinectomy. The natural ostium is enlarged firstly by lowering the mucosa onto the insertion of the inferior turbinate (e.g., with a microdebrider, as shown in ▶ Fig. 6.53, or an antrum punch); secondly through removal toward the posterior fontanelle (e.g., with straight through-cutting instruments, but keeping in mind the origin of the sphenopalatine artery); and finally, anteriorly toward the lacrimal crest (the surgeon should stop when he feels any resistance with the backbiting instrument, to avoid damage to the nasolacrimal apparatus).

This should allow the surgeon to evaluate an ample part of the maxillary sinus through angled endoscopes (30°/45° or up to 70°). However, the difficulties in maneuvering the dedicated curved and malleable instruments in a pure transnasal antral approach to the maxillary sinus must be always taken into consideration. The movement of curved tools to reach the alveolar recess under visualization with a 70° endoscope is definitely a technique that requires high levels of skill and experience and often requires a very large antrostomy.

It should be recognized, however, that even with angled endoscopes some areas of the alveolar recess are not visible through a transnasal approach, as illustrated in ▶ Fig. 6.54, and that the dedicated tools may fail to reach the more inferior and anterior regions of the maxillary sinus. In addition, there are no instruments able to cut bone or to exert a specific force in these spaces. For this reason, it is often necessary to combine transnasal and transoral approaches to achieve complete control of

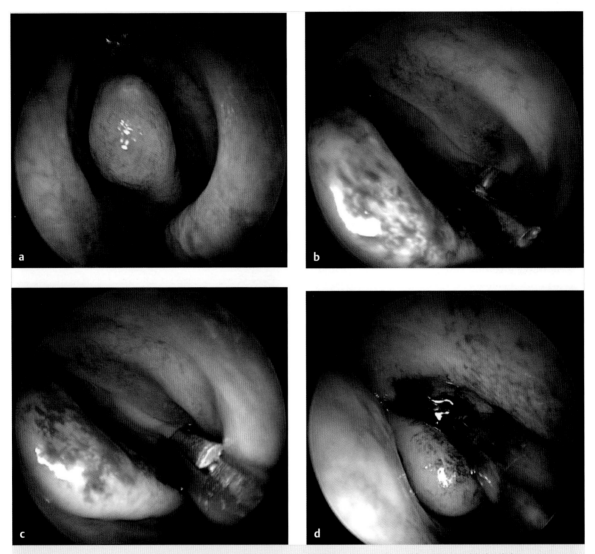

Fig. 6.50 Step-by-step uncinectomy. **(a)** Endoscopic view of the left middle turbinate. **(b)** Backbiter inserted behind the uncinate process right below the bulla floor. **(c)** Discharge of purulent material from the maxillary ostium. **(d)** Removal of the remaining middle part of the uncinate process with the microdebrider.

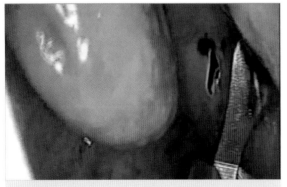

Fig. 6.51 Endoscopy of left accessory maxillary sinus ostium in the area of the fontanelles. The ostium lies completely in the sagittal plane.

the maxillary sinus within the inferior alveolar recess (▶ Fig. 6.55).

In patients with minor maxillary sinus disease the use of ballooning devices to dilate the ostium has been advocated (▶ Fig. 6.56). The limitations of this technique are, however, evident: no antrostomy is performed and no access to the sinus (with instruments) is gained.

Endoscopic Transnasal Anterior Approach to the Maxillary Sinus

This alternative approach may be useful in patients who need more anterior exposure and in patients for whom a combined oral approach is not indicated. Furthermore, this approach enables the surgeon to use 0° optics and

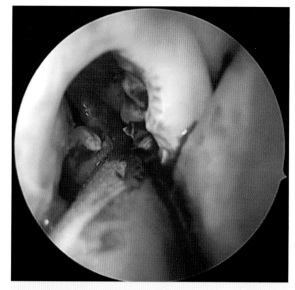

Fig. 6.52 Visualization of the right natural maxillary ostium after partial uncinectomy. The natural ostium is tilted horizontally with regards to the accessory ostium, which lies on a perfectly sagittal plane.

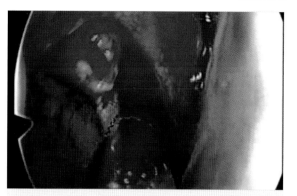

Fig. 6.53 Maxillary ostium enlarged with a microdebrider.

straight instruments to completely control the maxillary sinus.

In order to achieve an adequate exposure, this alternative involves entering the sinus through the inferior turbinate anteriorly to the lacrimal process, leaving the lacrimal duct intact: this approach is therefore indicated only when a deep lacrimal recess is present. For further

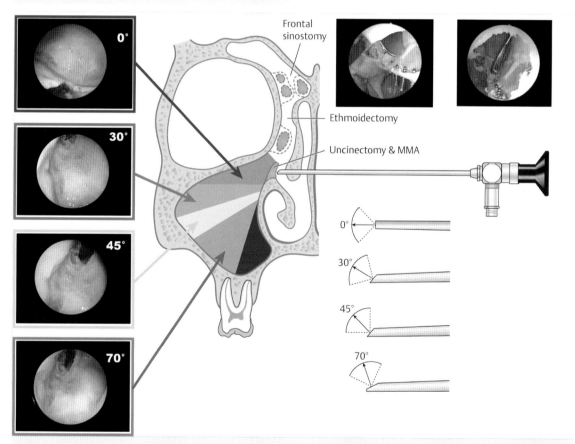

Fig. 6.54 (Left) View of the alveolar recess from a middle meatal antrostomy through different angled endoscopes (0–70°, color coded). **(Right)** Color-coded diagram showing visualization into the maxillary sinus. **(Top)** Accessibility of the alveolar recess with different angled instruments (with screws inserted to picture the seat of teeth), as seen from below through a canine fossa approach on a cadaver. Curved endoscopic forceps (upper right) inserted through the maxillary antrostomy are able to reach the floor of the sinus no further anterior than the third molar area (identified by the most posterior screw). Malleable instruments (upper left) inserted through the maxillary antrostomy can reach the floor of the sinus no further anterior than the second molar area (identified by the second most posterior screw). MMA, middle meatal antrostomy.

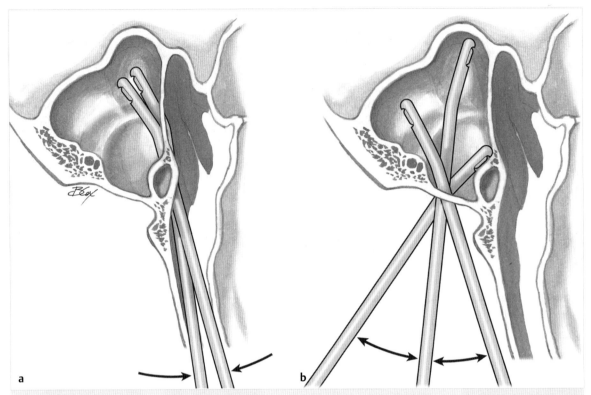

Fig. 6.55 (a) Microdebrider inserted through an antrostomy. Movement toward the anterior maxillary wall is greatly hindered by the nostrils and the anterior margin of the antrostomy. Only the posterior medial part of the sinus may be reached. **(b)** Microdebrider inserted through a canine fossa puncture. The whole maxillary sinus can be reached.

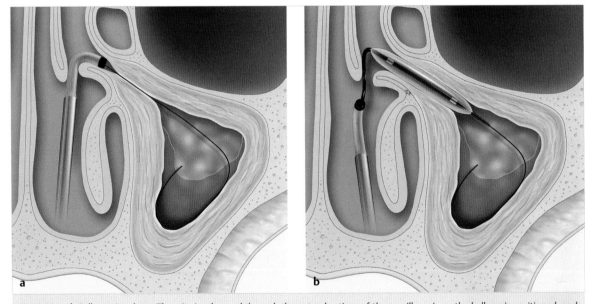

Fig. 6.56 a, b Balloon sinuplasty. The wire is advanced through the natural ostium of the maxillary sinus, the balloon is positioned, and the ostium is dilated via inflation.

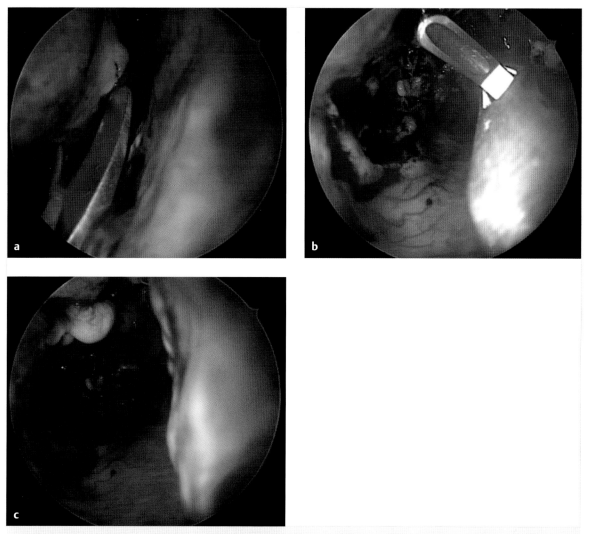

Fig. 6.57 Initial steps of right medial maxillectomy. **(a)** Incision behind the head of the inferior turbinate to remove its body and to try to conserve the lacrimal duct. **(b)** Inferior turbinate removed, and opening of the maxillary sinus through the inferior meatus. **(c)** Purulent discharge from the septate maxillary sinus.

references on this technique see the Manual of Endoscopic Sinus and Skull Base Surgery,[26]

Medial Maxillectomy

Often used for the surgical treatment of inverted papillomas or similar neoplastic diseases, the medial maxillectomy may also be indicated for a severely diseased maxillary sinus. As far as complications of dental treatments are concerned, this procedure is very useful in patients who have had several operations, especially those who have undergone previous open approaches such as the Caldwell–Luc procedure and present with major postoperative scarring, making conservative approaches to the sinus impossible, or in patients with partitioned sinuses.

The medial maxillectomy is based on the complete removal of the medial wall of the maxillary sinus, radical

removal of the inferior turbinate, and sometimes cutting of the nasolacrimal duct. The initial steps are illustrated in ▶ Fig. 6.57 a–c. This approach enables the endoscopic surgeon to reach all walls of the maxillary sinus with ease, apart from the anterior wall. For further references on the technique see Endoscopic Sinus Surgery.[25]

Ethmoidectomy

When the inflammatory and/or infectious process extends to the ethmoid, an anterior or even posterior ethmoidectomy may be advocated to clear all infectious secretions and to remove pathological edema of the mucosa that may lead to dysventilation of the neighboring sinuses.

As described in Chapter 1 (p.2), the ethmoid sinus is divided into an anterior and a posterior portion, with the

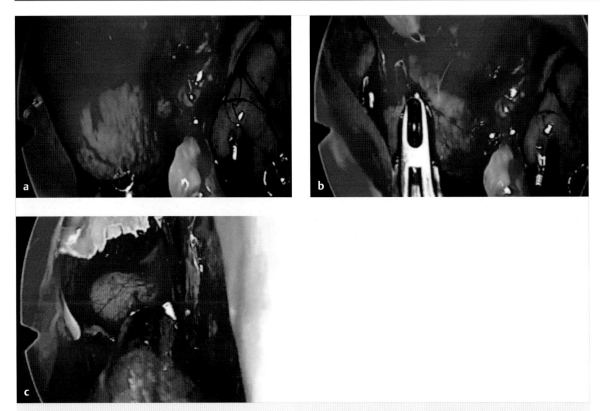

Fig. 6.58 Removal of the left ethmoidal bulla (a large antrostomy had already been performed). (a) Insertion of a curette into the lower medial part. (b) Removal of the anterior wall with through-cutting forceps. (c) Removal of the lateral walls with a microdebrider.

ethmoidal bulla and suprabullar cells being part of the anterior ethmoid, while the posterior ethmoid cells are found behind the ground lamella of the middle turbinate and medial and anterior to the lamella of the superior turbinate. In order to approach these sinuses, careful evaluation of the CT scans is needed, with identification of the ground lamella, the anterior and posterior ethmoidal arteries, the height and development of the skull base, and the assessment of any anatomical abnormality. Furthermore, thorough planning must be carried out, through identification on the CT scan of each cell or space that the surgeon wants to approach, to correlate imaging with the surgical view.

The first step is the opening of the inferomedial portion of the ethmoidal bulla. This may be achieved with a curette, a ball probe, or similar instrument that is slid medial to the anterior face of the bulla and then fractures its inferior part in order to remove the anterior wall, either with a microdebrider or with 45° Blakesley nasal forceps, as shown in ▶ Fig. 6.58 a–c. If only the anterior ethmoid requires opening, the surgeon may leave the borders of the cell untouched. Instead, if the surgeon must proceed with a posterior ethmoidectomy, removal of the whole cell is mandatory, in order to have good visibility and ample maneuverability (▶ Fig. 6.59).

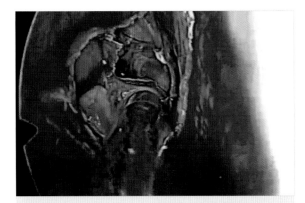

Fig. 6.59 Opening of anterior ethmoidal cells with a microdebrider.

The next step, when required, is to penetrate the ground lamella and sequentially remove all cells that have been identified on the CT scan. Due to possible anatomical variants of the ground lamella, the latter should always be perforated at an inferomedial site to avoid injury to the anterior skull base (▶ Fig. 6.60).

However, to ensure a safe removal, understanding of the transition between the posterior ethmoid and sphenoid is key and therefore, as already pointed out,

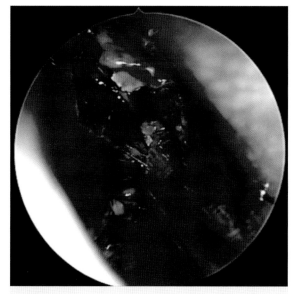

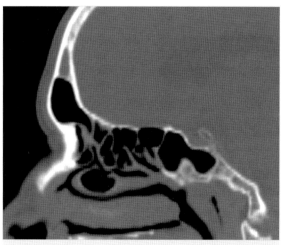

Fig. 6.61 Assessment of the ethmoid in a sagittal plain CT scan. The sphenoid sinus is an important landmark for the height of the skull base.

Fig. 6.60 Opening of the posterior ethmoid with a micro-debrider, through the basal lamella of the middle turbinate. Remnants of the bulla can be seen anteriorly.

thorough evaluation of the CT images is pivotal. Furthermore, a transnasal or transethmoidal approach to the sphenoid before complete removal of posterior cells may be very helpful, as the roof of the sphenoid can be used as a safe landmark for identification of the skull base (▶ Fig. 6.61).

Sphenoidal Sinusotomy/ Sphenoethmoidectomy

The sphenoid sinus can be approached either through its natural ostium via a direct transnasal route (e.g., for sinusitis limited to the sphenoid sinus) or, mainly when a posterior ethmoidectomy is also performed, through a transethmoidal sphenoidectomy.

When an approach to the sphenoid sinus is planned, the surgeon needs to check whether Onodi cells are present on CT scans, to visualize the anatomy of the patient's ethmoidal structures and the skull base height, as this is a key factor in performing a safe approach without the risk of harming the optic nerve or carotid artery or damaging the skull base.[1] However, if understanding the anatomy either during image evaluation or during surgery proves difficult, we suggest approaching the ostium first, in order to have a safe landmark from which to continue the surgical procedure.

- **Transnasal route** (via the sphenoethmoidal recess) (▶ Fig. 6.62a): The sphenoidal sinus can be safely found by reaching up from the posterior choana closely to the vomer with, for example, a curette or small straight sucker, as the ostium should lie approximately 10–15 mm above the border of the choana. An

additional landmark is the middle to lower third of the tail of the superior turbinate, as the ostium is usually located in close proximity and medially to it. However, a cautious lateralization of the middle turbinate may be necessary (e.g., with a Freer's elevator) to reach the ostium, as the turbinate body may hinder access to the sphenoethmoidal recess. As the anteromedial wall of the sinus is frequently very thin, a slight pressure is generally sufficient to enter into the sinus (always staying close to the vomer, to diminish the risk of entering the sinus and damaging the structures on the lateral wall (carotid artery and optic nerve). Once the surgeon has identified the ostium, its anterior wall can be removed up to the skull base (e.g., with a straight sphenoid punch or Hajek or Kerrison punch) (▶ Fig. 6.62b). However, in patients with inflammatory or infectious disease it is generally recommended that the ostium is enlarged by no more than one bite inferiorly, to avoid a lesion of the septal branch of the sphenopalatine artery.

- **Transethmoidal route** (▶ Fig. 6.62c): Following dissection of the posterior ethmoid cells, the sphenoid can be entered once the superior turbinate has been identified. First, the inferior part of this critical landmark is trimmed. A conservative removal (only the lower one-third) of the turbinate with straight through-cutting forceps enables the olfactory fibers to be preserved. Secondly, the border of the natural ostium is palpated, medial to the removed tail of the superior turbinate. It is worth noting that when the vomer is pneumatized or an Onodi cell is present, the ostium may be displaced laterally, medially, or downward. The anterior face of the sphenoid is then partially removed (e.g., with a Kerrison or Hajek punch). As already described, lowering of the opening may damage the septal branch of the sphenoidal artery and bipolar cautery may be necessary.

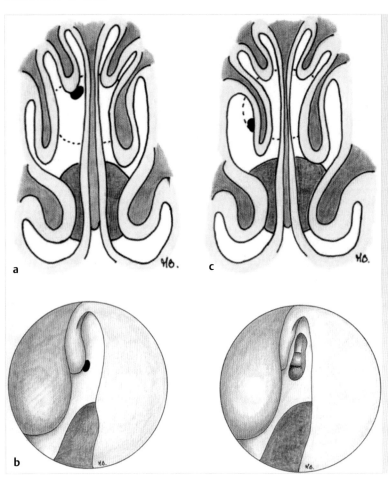

Fig. 6.62 Illustration of different approaches to the sphenoid sinus. **(a)** Access through the natural ostium in the sphenoethmoidal recess. **(b)** Close-up of the natural ostium and view into the sphenoid sinus after enlargement of the ostium. **(c)** Transethmoidal approach. (By kind permission of Dr. Manuela Bertazzoli.)

Finally, removal of the anterior face is extended laterally into the posterior ethmoid. This new opening should always be well below the optic nerve.

Surgical Approach to the Frontal Recess and Frontal Sinus

Frontal sinus surgery is considered by all endoscopic surgeons the most advanced and difficult step during training. Furthermore, this surgery is sometimes burdened with perioperative complications such as CSF leaks, ethmoidal artery lesions, and postoperative stenosis.

In patients with extramaxillary extension of odontogenic sinusitis, the need to approach the frontal sinus is rare and mostly confined to frontal recess surgery. More extensive frontal sinus surgery (median drainage procedures/DRAF III) is mainly indicated in patients with recurrent disease and in specific subsets of patients (ASA-syndrome, etc.), but these subjects are not addressed in this chapter. For further reading on median drainage procedures, see Endoscopic Sinus Surgery[25] or the Manual of Endoscopic Sinus and Skull Base Surgery.[26]

Whenever a patient presents with diffusion of infection from the maxillary sinus toward the frontal sinus, a frontal recess clearing is suggested. The assessment of the patient on a preoperative CT scan is fundamental for the successful removal of all cells that hinder complete drainage of the sinus into the meatus. A three-dimensional evaluation with axial, sagittal, and coronal scans is necessary to identify the drainage pathways to be cleared during surgery (▶ Fig. 6.63). The first step in such an assessment is the visualization of the agger nasi cell and the uncinate process. Moreover, identification of the frontal ethmoidal cells (type 1–4 in the modified Kuhn classification by Wormald[25]), frontal bulla cells, suprabullar cells, and intersinus septal cells, is necessary to achieve successful clearing.

Once the drainage pathway has been identified on CT scans, the surgeon removes the cells sequentially (e.g., using a frontal sinus probe or frontal curette), exposing the frontal sinus ostium. In order to reach these cells the surgeon follows the cranial part of the uncinate process and removes it up to its attachment with a 45° through-cutting forceps. Sometimes, a transaxillary access (removal of the anterior wall of the agger nasi cell with a Hajek punch with/without raising of a mucoperiosteal axillary

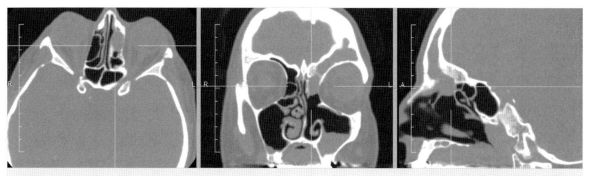

Fig. 6.63 Frontal sinus surgery planning: CT scan in three planes, allowing three-dimensional assessment of the frontal drainage pathway.

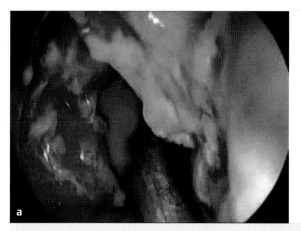
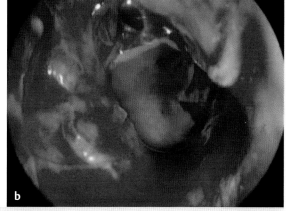

Fig. 6.64 (a) Opened frontal sinus. **(b)** A different perspective.

flap) may ease this approach. The surgeon should then have good vision (with a 45° endoscope) of the remaining cells that block the drainage pathway, and these are removed by sliding a frontal curette or a probe medially toward the middle turbinate and rupturing them in a lateral direction (▶ Fig. 6.64 a, b). Preservation of the mucosa, draping it on the lateral nasal wall, and removal of the bony shells of the cells are of paramount importance. Finally, careful palpation will confirm if all cells have been removed according to the preoperative three-dimensional assessment.

Management of Anatomical Anomalies of the Middle Turbinate

The middle turbinate may be paradoxically curved and this significantly narrows the passageway to the middle meatus, consequently reducing ventilation and drainage of the maxillary, frontal, and ethmoid sinuses. Furthermore, this abnormality may hinder an efficient approach to the uncinate process and the anterior or posterior ethmoid. If indicated, a paradoxically bent middle turbinate should be corrected, according to the extent of the

obstruction, by means of a partial turbinoplasty of the turbinate head with through-cutting straight and 45° nasal forceps.

Likewise, a heavily pneumatized middle turbinate, called a concha bullosa, may compromise the ventilation and drainage of the ostiomeatal complex. In a patient with symptomatic obstruction, incision of the turbinate head with a scalpel and partial resection of the lateral aspect of the concha bullosa with curved and/or straight nasal scissors may be indicated (▶ Fig. 6.65). This procedure will correct the shape of the middle turbinate and improve ventilation.

Endoscopic and Traditional Septoplasty

The surgical correction of a septal spur or deviation, unless it is responsible for respiratory obstruction or blockage of the middle meatus, may be indicated only if it represents an obstacle to the use of endoscopic or traditional instruments.

In patients with an isolated septal ridge or spur, a mucosal incision is made with a scalpel, sickle knife, or angled round knife along the deviation. The incision can be performed either horizontally or vertically in front of the deviation, creating a U-shaped flap. The mucosa cranial and caudal to the spur is elevated and an incision of the cartilage to raise the mucosa of the contralateral side is performed with a Freer elevator or suction Freer. If correctly performed, the perichondrium should remain intact and adherent to the mucosa on both sides. The next step is to isolate the deviation and to remove its osteocartilaginous elements with Blakesley forceps and/or osteotomes. Normally, the flaps readily adhere to the intact contralateral side and no suture positioning is necessary to cover the defect (▶ Fig. 6.66 a, b).

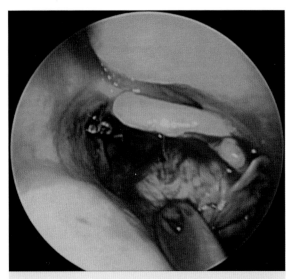

Fig. 6.65 Turbinoplasty of a right concha bullosa (removal of its lateral part).

When the septal deviation is very anterior or involves the whole septum, a traditional septoplasty under endoscopic visualization with a monolateral or bilateral anterior transfixing incision may be indicated (▶ Fig. 6.67). This procedure can be performed very precisely using endoscopy. If correctly performed, the traditional septoplasty is very well tolerated by the patient, with minimal postoperative discomfort, and can be associated with any other endoscopic transnasal technique or with transoral approaches.

Management of Other Anatomical Anomalies

The nose and paranasal sinuses can present other anatomical abnormalities, such as Haller cells (an ethmoidal cell partially closing the ostium of the maxillary sinus) or Onodi cells (an ethmoidal cell partially posterior to the sphenoid sinus). Onodi cells should always be identified on CT scans when planning approaches to the sphenoid and posterior ethmoid, as the surgeon may lose reference points and damage the optic nerve, which is located within or close to its lateral wall, if not dehiscent. Where Haller cells are present, however, as long as they do not hinder the ventilation and drainage of the paranasal cavities, no surgical removal is needed. On the contrary, if Haller cells are clinically symptomatic or are likely to block the maxillary ostium in the postoperative period, they must be opened and removed using an endoscopic approach (i.e., with Heuwieser antrum forceps), following enlargement of the natural ostium.

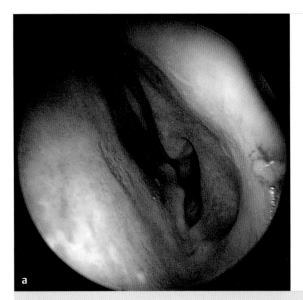
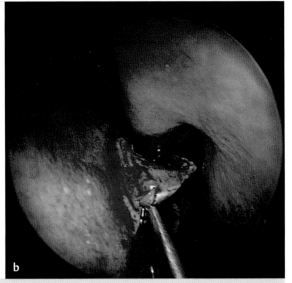

Fig. 6.66 Endoscopic septoplasty. **(a)** View of left septal spur after decongestion. **(b)** Removal of the deviated septum after incision of the septal mucosa.

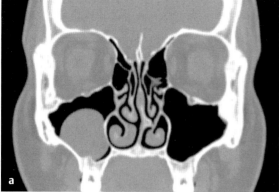

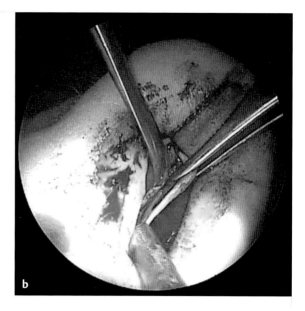

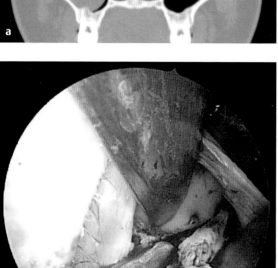

Fig. 6.67 Traditional septoplasty. **(a)** CT scan of left-deviated septum. **(b)** Elevation of the mucoperichondrium. **(c)** Removal of the deviated septal cartilage.

6.2.3 Transnasal Surgical Approach to Complications of Dental Disease and Treatment

Management of Dental Complications Pertaining to the Maxillary Sinus

Depending on the timespan between displacement of the foreign body into the maxillary sinus and patient consultation, the disruption of sinus homeostasis and therefore the infectious involvement may be more pronounced and the planned approach more extensive. The choice of the correct approach is therefore guided by the extent of infection, if present. Intuitively, the first step is the localization of the foreign body via maxillofacial CT imaging.

Because the foreign materials may change their positions over time due to mucociliary clearance, a radiographic re-evaluation (e.g., panoramic radiograph) no more than 24 hours prior to surgery is strongly recommended. Radiographs will show if the foreign body is located directly on the sinus floor or near the maxillary ostium: this information will guide the extent of the approach to the ostium. The second step is the assessment of maxillary sinus involvement by means of imaging and endoscopy: opacification of the sinus on CT scans and purulent discharge in the middle meatus are the relevant findings. An additional sign of the severity of maxillary sinus infection is the anteriorization of the uncinate process, as this corresponds to a high-pressure process inside the sinus combined with its isolation from the nasal cavity (▶ Fig. 6.68).

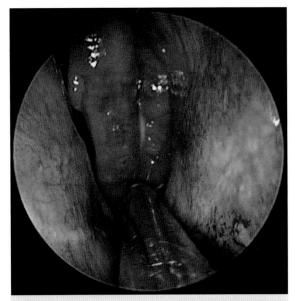

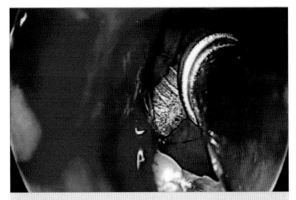

Fig. 6.69 Endoscopic removal of an implant displaced into the maxillary sinus through an intranasal middle meatal antrostomy.

Fig. 6.68 Anteriorization of the left uncinate process with purulent discharge coming out of the middle meatus.

As described in Section 6.3.2 (p. 104), Surgical Techniques, the maxillary sinus can be approached in a variety of ways; however, the most frequent approach is performed with an enlargement of the maxillary natural ostium after uncinectomy. See the earlier section on Antrostomy for a step-by-step guide. The use of angled optics (30°, 45°, 70°) and curved instruments will ease the removal (▶ Fig. 6.69). Often, pressure-irrigation with saline through curved aspirators may help the movement of particularly "stubborn" bodies. In patients with foreign bodies and no maxillary sinus infection, the antrostomy size should be as small as possible and mainly determined by the size of the foreign body to be removed. However, materials located exclusively in the alveolar recess may be hard to reach transnasally and it is preferable, in patients with no sinusal infection, to adopt an oral approach (canine fossa/antral retriever). See ▶ Table 6.1 and Section 6.2.2 (p. 86) for details of endoscopic oral approaches.

In patients with displaced material in the maxillary sinus and concomitant maxillary sinusitis, antrostomy for removal of the foreign body is almost always sufficient to simultaneously treat the sinus infection. However, we advocate sinusal irrigation with either saline alone or saline plus 30% H_2O_2 (▶ Fig. 6.70) to remove the purulent secretions from the mucosa. If an extramucosal fungal infection (fungus ball) is present, these irrigations may also ease the complete removal of the fungal material (fungus ball mostly consists of very brittle caseous material and may at

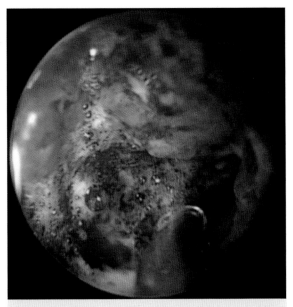

Fig. 6.70 H_2O_2 lavage of the maxillary sinus after antrostomy.

times be difficult to remove with grasping instruments) (▶ Fig. 6.71 a–d).

Rinsing the maxillary sinus is also helpful in classic odontogenic sinusitis of the maxillary sinus without foreign body displacement.

Whenever the infection involves other paranasal sinuses, these should be addressed at the same time as the removal of the foreign body. Please refer to Section 6.3.2 (p. 104) for step-by-step guides to ethmoidectomy, sphenoidal sinusotomy, and frontal sinus surgery. While approaching the other paranasal sinuses (▶ Fig. 6.72), the surgeon must bear in mind that it is only necessary to obtain good drainage, as the source of infection has already been removed.

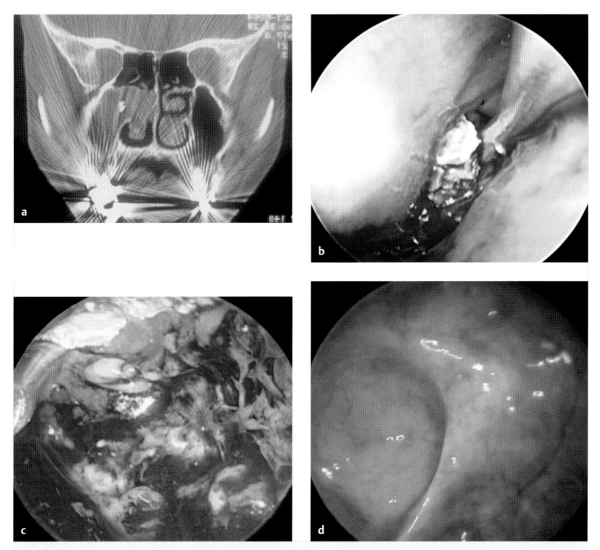

Fig. 6.71 Maxillary fungus ball. **(a)** CT scan of a right maxillary fungus ball, with pathognomonic ironlike sign on the scan. **(b)** Removal of the friable formation. **(c)** Maxillary sinus after partial removal. **(d)** Endoscopic follow-up at 40 days.

Management of Complications Pertaining to the Other Paranasal Sinuses and Nasal Fossae

In the following paragraphs the surgical approach to the removal of teeth/roots or implants displaced or migrated into the other paranasal sinuses and the nasal fossae will be detailed.

As in all patients with migrated materials, a radiographic re-evaluation (e.g., panoramic radiograph) no more than 24 hours prior to surgery is strongly recommended. In the patient with displaced material in the nasal fossae, a simple endoscopic exploration (with 0° or 30° endoscopes under local anesthesia) combined with the use of nasal forceps (Blakesley straight or upturned), may be enough to remove implants or other foreign bodies (▸ Fig. 6.73 a, b). In the patient with displaced material in the ethmoid or sphenoid sinus or the frontal recess, local anesthesia may be insufficient to allow the safe removal of a foreign body. Endoscopy under general anesthesia may be a better approach in case deeper parts of the sinuses need to be accessed.

After removal of the foreign body, a thorough evaluation of the integrity of the skull base in patients with displaced implants in the upper sphenoid sinus or frontal recess is strongly recommended.

Finally, a simple trick to use when implants do not easily come out of the nasal lining is to turn them counterclockwise, as, due to the ciliary action and the intrinsic properties of the screws, these tend to self-tap into the mucosa and bone.

6.2.4 Clinical Cases (History, Imaging, Treatment, Outcome)

Transnasal Approach: Case 1

▶ Fig. 6.74 a–g shows the case of a patient suffering from maxillary sinusitis with an implant displaced into the right maxillary sinus.

The patient, a 62-year-old man, underwent two dental implants positioned in his upper jaw. The left implant integrated into the bone. The right implant dislocated into the maxillary sinus a few days after positioning due to lack of adequate bone height. The patient didn't notice the dislocation of the implant, but developed signs and symptoms of sinusitis within a month of dental implant

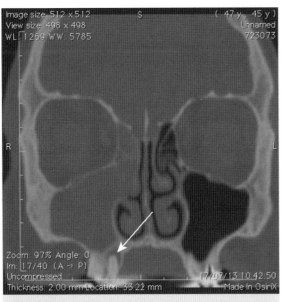

Fig. 6.72 Extramaxillary extension of odontogenic sinusitis into the ethmoid. A periapical infection (*arrow*) is the source of the infection.

positioning. He underwent an ENT consultation, and during imaging examination, the implant was identified and an endoscopic treatment was planned.

Transnasal Approach: Case 2

The case of a patient with an implant displaced into the sphenoid sinus in shown in ▶ Fig. 6.75 a–c. The patient, a 43-year-old woman, was referred to the ENT department by her dentist after the whole dental implant along with its coupler were displaced into the maxillary sinus during the dental procedure. Seven days passed before the ENT consultation, and by then the implant had left the maxillary sinus via the natural ostium and reached the sphenoid sinus. An endoscopic procedure under general anesthesia was planned.

6.2.5 Classification Example

When a patient undergoes several dental treatments ranging from maxillary sinus augmentation to implantology and dental extractions, classification can be difficult. A case of complex classification is hereby provided, where the patient shows signs of prior maxillary sinus augmentation, oroantral communication and dental implants placement. Example of a classification is shown in ▶ Fig. 6.76 a–b.

> **Key Points**
>
> - How to approach the ostia of the paranasal sinuses transnasally.
> - How to manage maxillary, ethmoidal, frontal, and sphenoidal sinusitis endoscopically.
> - How to manage foreign bodies displaced/migrated into the maxillary sinus or other paranasal sinuses.
> - Advantages and disadvantages of transnasal endoscopic approaches.

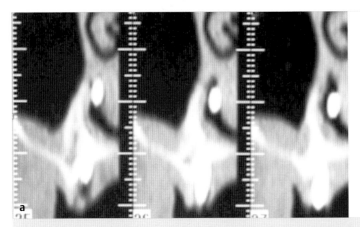
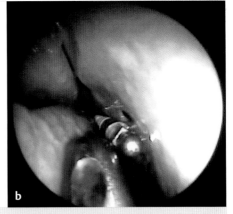

Fig. 6.73 (a) Dental scan of migrated implant in the inferior meatus. (b) Removal of the implant under local anesthesia.

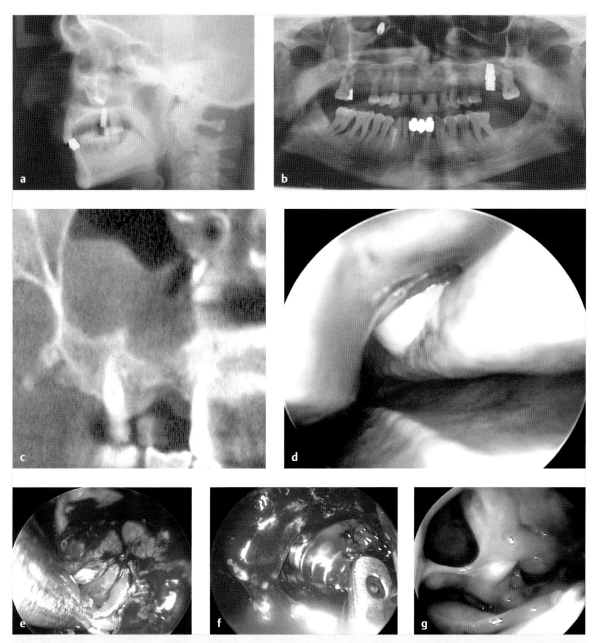

Fig. 6.74 Patient suffering from recurrent acute right maxillary sinus infection. **(a–c)** Imaging showing an implant displaced into the right maxillary sinus with right maxillary sinus infection. The orthopantomography was taken 4 hours prior to surgery to check the position of the implant. **(d–f)** Exclusive transnasal surgical approach: purulent discharge in the middle meatus; opening of the maxillary sinus through a middle meatal antrostomy with visualization of hyperplastic mucosa of the maxillary sinus; and removal of the displaced implant with a grasping forceps. **(g)** Endoscopic follow-up at 40 days.

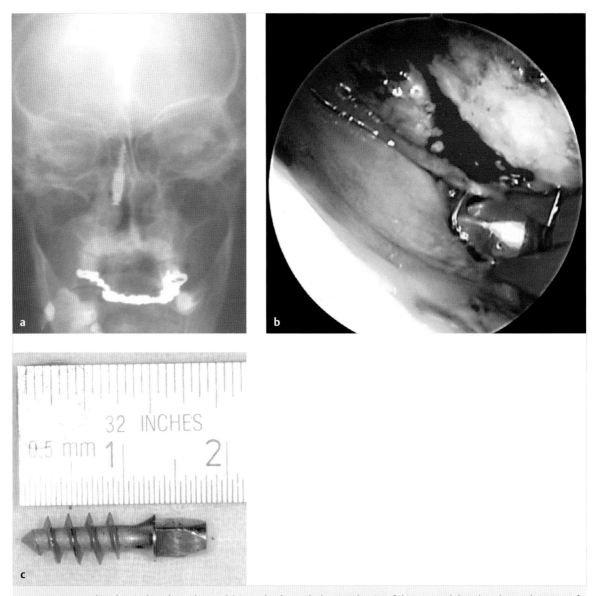

Fig. 6.75 Migrated implant in the sphenoid sinus. **(a)** Frontal radiograph showing the site of the migrated dental implant and no signs of sinusal inflammation. **(b)** Removal of the implant from the anterior wall of the sphenoid sinus was difficult as it self-tapped into the bone. **(c)** Implant.

6.3 Multidisciplinary Approach (Endoscopic and Intraoral)

6.3.1 Introduction

As already described, an endoscopic approach via a transnasal access (FESS, functional endoscopic sinus surgery) can successfully be used for the removal of foreign bodies from the paranasal sinuses, whether the patient is affected by sinusitis or not.[27–30] However, it must be emphasized that this technique, which on the one hand

preserves the integrity of the maxillary sinus walls and of the sinus mucosa, does on the other hand present some limitations.

The first is related to the removal of foreign bodies located in the anterior and inferior part of the maxillary sinus. This area is difficult to reach via a transnasal access with the endoscopic instruments currently available. The second limitation is that with FESS it is impossible to remove infected roots/teeth or implants penetrating into the sinus but still embedded in the alveolar bone. The third limitation is that FESS does not allow closure of oroantral communications.

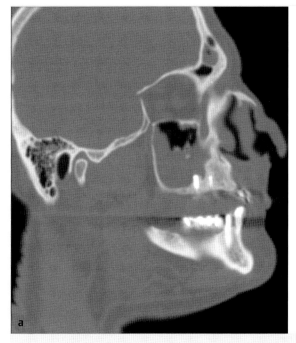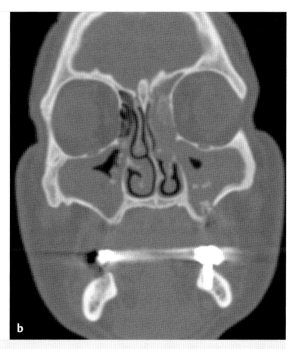

Fig. 6.76 (a, b) Classification example: sagittal and coronal CT scans depicting a patient with bilateral sinusitis after bilateral sinus lift procedure and implant placement (note the migrated grafting material in both maxillary sinuses). Following the flow chart simplifies the classification into class 1a, although the patient underwent different treatments (both implant-related and augmentation-related).

FESS is therefore a first-choice procedure in patients with foreign bodies displaced into the maxillary sinus, in particular if a significant sinus infection or inflammatory reaction of the sinus mucosa and an ostium obstruction are present, and/or other paranasal sinuses are involved in the infection.[30]

In such patients, it is possible in one single session to access the maxillary sinus and all the other paranasal sinuses (if involved) with the aim of removing foreign bodies and all the infected material and also improving the drainage and ventilation of the paranasal sinuses.

In contrast, if there is no significant sinus infection, the ostium is not obstructed by inflammatory reaction of the sinus mucosa, the other paranasal sinuses do not show any inflammatory or infectious reaction (despite the presence of a foreign body), an intraoral approach (a Caldwell–Luc operation, using the pedicled bony window technique or an intraoral endoscopic approach) seems to be an excellent alternative. It is also worth noting that the presence of an oroantral communication renders an intraoral approach the only technique available.

It must also be noted that, in patients with a moderate sinus mucosal reaction, sinus anatomy and function normally return to a healthy state once the foreign body is removed, as demonstrated in several studies.[6,29,30]

Conversely, if significant infection is present involving the maxillary sinus and/or other paranasal sinuses, the maxillary sinus ostium is obstructed, an oroantral communication is present, and, finally, foreign bodies are located in the anterior/inferior corner of the maxillary sinus (not all of these factors need necessarily be present at the same time), a combination of FESS and an intraoral approach seems to be the best choice available.

6.3.2 Techniques

The technical details of FESS and intraoral approaches have been already described. In this section, only the specific features of the combined approach will be examined.

Due to the dual approach and the longer operating time, the combined procedure is normally performed under general anesthesia. This allows a controlled blood hypotension to be maintained, with reduction of bleeding, which is particularly useful in the endoscopic phase. An orotracheal intubation is performed to leave free access to the nasal cavities, in particular when paranasal sinuses are involved on both sides.

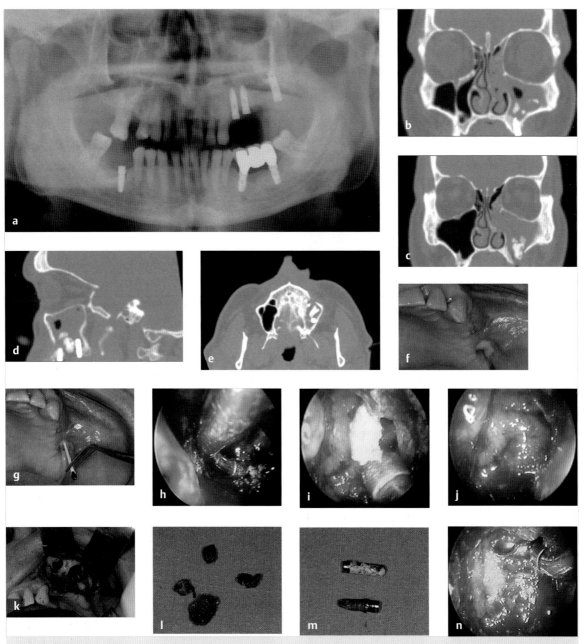

Fig. 6.77 **(a)** Panoramic radiograph showing three implants in place and an irregular opacity of the maxillary sinus. **(b,c)** Coronal CT scans demonstrating the penetration of the apical portion of an implant into the maxillary sinus and some biomaterial aggregates dispersed inside the sinusal lumen. The maxillary sinus appears completely opacified, as are the ipsilateral ethmoidal cells. **(d,e)** Sagittal and axial CT scans demonstrating the penetration of two implants into the sinusal lumen, the dispersed biomaterial, and the diffuse sinusal opacity. **(f,g)** Spontaneous pus discharge in the area of the most distal implant; the presence of an oroantral fistula is assessed with the aid of a sterile gutta-percha cone. **(h,i)** Once access to the maxillary sinus is gained via a transnasal endoscopic approach, it is possible to visualize and remove the infected biomaterial (in the form of small granules or large aggregates) dispersed into the sinus lumen, by means of suction and dedicated instruments. **(j)** After removal of the dispersed biomaterial and a thorough curettage, the sinusal cavity is visually checked to ensure that no biomaterial particles are left in areas of the sinus that are not accessible from the intraoral access. **(k)** After elevation of a full-thickness flap and removal of the implants protruding into the sinus lumen, the extent of maxillary bone loss is visible. **(l,m)** The removed residual biomaterial particles and implants. **(n)** The oroantral communication is demonstrated by the endoscopic view (via an intranasal postantrostomy approach) of a surgical curette inserted into the bony defect exposed by the intraoral access.

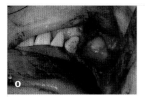
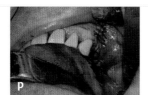
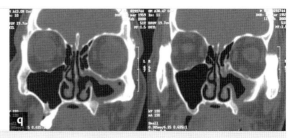

Fig. 6.77 (*Continued*) **(o,p)** Owing to the extent of maxillary bone loss, a fat pad flap is used to act as a supporting layer for the overlying Rehrmann flap, to avoid postoperative dehiscence of the surgical wound. **(q)** Coronal CT scan demonstrating resolution of the maxillary and ethmoidal sinusitis.

The surgical procedure starts with the endoscopic phase. Uncinectomy and reduction of the middle turbinate (if indicated) ease the access to the maxillary sinus ostium, which is enlarged to improve access to the sinus. Displaced foreign bodies can be removed from the maxillary sinus in this phase, unless they are inaccessible owing to their position in the anterior /inferior recess of the sinus or they are still integrated into the bone. In this latter case, removal of the foreign body is performed during the intraoral phase. Cautious removal of hyperplastic/polypoid mucosa can be undertaken, taking care to preserve the remaining nonpathological maxillary sinus mucosa.

It is possible to access the other paranasal sinuses (if involved in the infection) during the same session and to remove all the infectious material, hyperplastic/polypoid mucosa, and, finally, foreign bodies such as implants that have migrated into them. By opening the ethmoidal cells and/or the frontal/sphenoidal ostium, it is possible to accelerate the recovery of paranasal sinus function.

The second phase consists of the intraoral approach, which allows removal of foreign bodies located in parts of the maxillary sinus not easily accessible via the endoscopic approach (in particular, the anterior/inferior part) or removal of teeth/roots responsible for sinus infection but still embedded in the alveolar bone. At the end of surgery, just prior to closure of the oroantral communication (if present), it is possible to inspect the sinus with endoscopes from both the intraoral and the intranasal approaches, thereby reducing the chances of leaving behind remnants of foreign bodies or infected material.

6.3.3 Clinical Cases (History, Imaging, Treatment, Outcome)

Combined Approach: Case 1

The patient, a 48-year-old man, underwent a sinus floor elevation and grafting procedure in association with the placement of three endosseous implants. The treatment had been provided in a private dental practice 6 months previously, and since the date of the intervention the patient had complained of symptoms such as swelling, fluid discharge into the nasal cavity, pus discharge into the oral cavity, and a sense of heaviness and discomfort in the maxillary region. Antibiotic therapy based on penicillin and a chlorhexidine mouthwash regimen was administered but the symptoms did not regress. For this reason, the patient decided to consult another specialist and came to our attention. The case is illustrated in ▶ Fig. 6.77 a–q.

Combined Approach: Case 2

The patient, a 55-year-old woman, had received a blade-type implant in the upper left posterior maxilla 5 years previously, to support a fixed bridge. The prosthetic rehabilitation became loose and other symptoms, such as nasal discharge and soreness in the maxillary region, began to develop. For these reasons the patient sought a specialist's advice and came to our attention. The case is illustrated in ▶ Fig. 6.78 a–n.

Key Points

- A combined approach can solve in the same surgical session sinonasal pathologies associated with odontogenic sinusitis that cannot be treated with an intraoral approach (infection involving the frontal, ethmoidal, sphenoidal sinuses, maxillary ostium obstruction).
- A combined approach can eliminate problems not treatable using an endoscopic approach (removal of infected teeth or implants still embedded in alveolar bone, removal of foreign bodies located in the anterior/inferior recess of the maxillary sinus not accessible via a FESS approach, closure of oroantral communications).

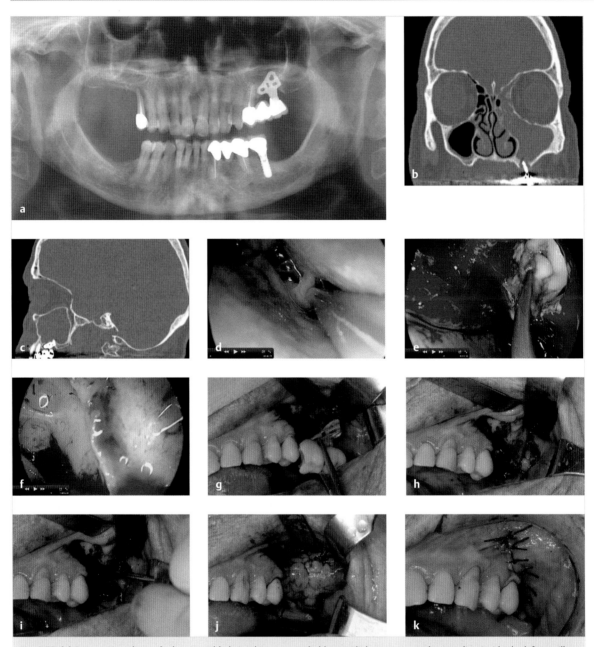

Fig. 6.78 **(a)** Panoramic radiograph showing a blade implant surrounded by a radiolucent area and protruding inside the left maxillary sinus. **(b,c)** Coronal and sagittal CT scans showing the loss of integration of the implant, the loss of alveolar bone, and a radiopacity involving the entire lumen of the maxillary sinus and some ethmoidal cells. **(d,e)** Endoscopic stills showing the presence of purulent material in the nasal cavity and inside the maxillary sinus. **(f)** The purulent material is eliminated and the maxillary sinus is irrigated with sterile saline; the endoscopic phase has been completed. **(g)** The intraoral phase begins with the separation of the prosthetic bridge, the elevation of a full-thickness flap, and the removal of the blade implant. **(h,i)** The extent of the bone loss is now visible, and the area around the oroantral communication is treated with a thorough curettage and irrigation with sterile saline to eliminate all remaining infected tissue and purulent material. **(j,k)** A buccal fat pad flap is sutured to the palatal side of the surgical access, forming a stable base layer for the overlying Rehrmann flap, which is repositioned with water-tight sutures.

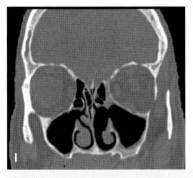 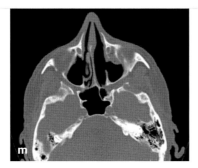 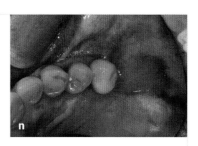

Fig. 6.78 (*Continued*) **(l,m)** Coronal and axial CT scans showing the complete resolution of the ethmoidal and maxillary sinusitis. **(n)** One month after suture removal it is possible to verify the complete healing of the soft tissues.

References

[1] Kim H-U, Kim SS, Kang SS, Chung IH, Lee JG, Yoon JH. Surgical anatomy of the natural ostium of the sphenoid sinus. Laryngoscope 2001; 111: 1599–1602

[2] Caldwell G. Diseases of the accessory sinuses of the nose and an improved method of treatment for suppuration of the maxillary antrum. N Y Med J 1893; 58: 526–528

[3] Hasegawa J, Watanabe K, Kunitomo M et al. Foreign body in the maxillary sinus—possible plastic tube: a case report. Auris Nasus Larynx 2003; 30: 299–301

[4] Sahin YF, Muderris T, Bercin S, Sevil E, Kiris M. Chronic maxillary sinusitis associated with an unusual foreign body: a case report. Case Rep Otolaryngol 2012; 2012: 903714

[5] Biglioli F, Goisis M. Access to the maxillary sinus using a bone flap on a mucosal pedicle: preliminary report. J Craniomaxillofac Surg 2002; 30: 255–259

[6] Biglioli F, Chiapasco M. An easy access to retrieve dental implants displaced into the maxillary sinus: the bony window technique. Clin Oral Implants Res 2014; 25: 1344–1351

[7] Mantovani M, Pipolo C, Messina F, Felisati G, Torretta S, Pignataro L. Antral retriever and displaced dental implants in the maxillary sinus. J Craniofac Surg 2011; 22: 2275–2277

[8] Nakamura N, Mitsuyasu T, Ohishi M. Endoscopic removal of a dental implant displaced into the maxillary sinus: technical note. Int J Oral Maxillofac Surg 2004; 33: 195–197

[9] Pfeifer G. Über Ursachen von neuralgiformen Schmerzen nach Kieferhöhlenoperationen und Möglichkeiten der chirurgischen Behandlung. Dtsch Zahn Mund Kieferheilkd 1973; 60: 201–213

[10] Penttilä MA, Rautiainen ME, Pukander JS, Karma PH. Endoscopic versus Caldwell-Luc approach in chronic maxillary sinusitis: comparison of symptoms at one-year follow-up. Rhinology 1994; 32: 161–165

[11] Stammberger H, Zinreich SJ, Kopp W, Kennedy DW, Johns ME, Rosenbaum AE. Surgical treatment of chronic recurrent sinusitis—the Caldwell-Luc versus a functional endoscopic technic [in German] HNO 1987; 35: 93–105

[12] Stammberger H. History of rhinology: anatomy of the paranasal sinuses. Rhinology 1989; 27: 197–210

[13] Kessler P, Hardt N. The use of micro-titanium mesh for maxillary sinus wall reconstruction. J Craniomaxillofac Surg 1996; 24: 317–321

[14] Laskin D, Dierks E. Diagnosis and treatment of diseases and disorders of the maxillary sinus. Oral Maxillofac Surg Clin North Am 1999; 11: 1–183

[15] Lindorf HH. Osteoplastic surgery of the sinus maxillaris—the "bone lid"-method. J Maxillofac Surg 1984; 12: 271–276

[16] Widmark G, Ekholm S, Borrman H, Grangård U, Holmberg K. The use of a bone lid to close the anterior wall defect after surgery in the maxillary sinus. Swed Dent J 1992; 16: 173–182

[17] Choi BH, Yoo JH, Sung KJ. Radiographic comparison of osseous healing after maxillary sinusotomy performed with and without a periosteal pedicle. Oral Surg Oral Med Oral Pathol Oral Radiol Endod 1996; 82: 375–378

[18] Stammberger H. Functional Endoscopic Sinus Surgery: The Messerklinger Technique. St Louis, MO: Mosby-Year Book; 1991:283–289

[19] Barrault S. Dental infections and sinoscopy [in French]. Rev Stomatol Chir Maxillofac 1985; 86: 386–388

[20] Joe Jacob K, George S, Preethi S, Arunraj VS. A comparative study between endoscopic middle meatal antrostomy and caldwell-luc surgery in the treatment of chronic maxillary sinusitis. Indian J Otolaryngol Head Neck Surg 2011; 63: 214–219

[21] Lee JY, Lee SH, Hong HS, Lee JD, Cho SH. Is the canine fossa puncture approach really necessary for the severely diseased maxillary sinus during endoscopic sinus surgery? Laryngoscope 2008; 118: 1082–1087

[22] Giovannetti F, Priore P, Raponi I, Valentini V. Endoscopic sinus surgery in sinus-oral pathology. J Craniofac Surg 2014; 25: 991–994

[23] Ahn HJ, Chung SK, Dhong HJ et al. Comparison of surgical conditions during propofol or sevoflurane anaesthesia for endoscopic sinus surgery. Br J Anaesth 2008; 100: 50–54

[24] Schlosser RJ, Spotnitz WD, Peters EJ, Fang K, Gaston B, Gross CW. Elevated nitric oxide metabolite levels in chronic sinusitis. Otolaryngol Head Neck Surg 2000; 123: 357–362

[25] Wormald PJ. Endoscopic Sinus Surgery: Anatomy, Three-Dimensional Reconstruction, and Surgical Technique. 3rd ed. Thieme; 2013

[26] Simmen D, Jones N. Manual of Endoscopic Sinus and Skull Base Surgery. 2nd ed. Thieme; 2013

[27] Iida S, Tanaka N, Kogo M, Matsuya T. Migration of a dental implant into the maxillary sinus. A case report. Int J Oral Maxillofac Surg 2000; 29: 358–359

[28] Kitamura A. Removal of a migrated dental implant from a maxillary sinus by transnasal endoscopy. Br J Oral Maxillofac Surg 2007; 45: 410–411

[29] Felisati G, Lozza P, Chiapasco M, Borloni R. Endoscopic removal of an unusual foreign body in the sphenoid sinus: an oral implant. Clin Oral Implants Res 2007; 18: 776–780

[30] Chiapasco M, Felisati G, Maccari A, Borloni R, Gatti F, Di Leo F. The management of complications following displacement of oral implants in the paranasal sinuses: a multicenter clinical report and proposed treatment protocols. Int J Oral Maxillofac Surg 2009; 38: 1273–1278

Chapter 7

ENT Contraindications to Maxillary Sinus Grafting Prior To or In Association with Oral Implant Placement

7

7 ENT Contraindications to Maxillary Sinus Grafting Prior To or In Association with Oral Implant Placement

Giovanni Felisati, Alberto Maria Saibene, Matteo Chiapasco, Sara Torretta, Lorenzo Pignataro

Contents Overview

This chapter will deal with the complex relationship between maxillary sinus grafting and sinonasal cavities. First, a brief overview is provided of the pathophysiological mechanisms underlying the development of sinonasal complications after maxillary sinus grafting. The chapter then focuses on the ear, nose, and throat (ENT) contraindications to this procedure, taking into account which contraindications should be considered reversible and which irreversible. Lastly, a complete reference is given on the treatment options for reversible contraindications.

7.1 Introduction

Maxillary sinus grafting (MSG, also known as maxillary sinus elevation or sinus lift) is a successful procedure with predictable outcomes, which has been routinely performed for more than 30 years to allow the placement of oral implants for the subsequent prosthetic restoration of atrophic and edentulous posterior maxillae.[1]

Although MSG modifies the local anatomy of the maxillary sinus and may temporarily impair sinus homeostasis, due to the surgical trauma that may induce inflammatory periosteal swelling or reduced ciliary activity, it has been demonstrated that initially "healthy" sinuses with adequate ciliary clearance and patent ostia recover very rapidly in the vast majority of patients.[2] As a matter of fact, despite the anatomical modifications following sinus floor elevation procedures, the occurrence of sinus-related complications after MSG, if properly performed, is generally low (<4%), as reported in the literature.[1,3–7]

On the other hand, potential candidates for MSG procedures presenting with preexisting impaired anatomical and functional conditions of the sinuses (such as a history of chronic sinusitis) may be exposed to an increased incidence of sinus-related complications,[1,5,6,8–12] as an already "unhealthy" sinus may not tolerate or recover properly from an MSG procedure. Although no controlled clinical trials have been performed to assess the correlation between the incidence of complications following MSG and the initial anatomo-physiological status of the maxillary sinus, it is reasonable to speculate that the success rate of the procedure could be partially related to the baseline anatomo-physiological conditions: the better the starting condition of the sinus, the lower the risk of complications. It is therefore mandatory to perform a thorough preoperative evaluation of the initial condition of the maxillary sinus before planning an MSG procedure.

7.2 Evaluation of the Candidate for Maxillary Sinus Elevation

Before performing an MSG, every oral surgeon should carefully evaluate the patient by collecting a detailed case history and conducting proper radiological tests. Any condition that may jeopardize maxillary sinus drainage and ventilation must be detected, as it might predispose the patient to the development of sinus-related complications after the surgical procedure. If any risk to maxillary sinus homeostasis is discovered, the patient should be referred to an ENT surgeon to perform a thorough ENT evaluation, including nasal endoscopy, in order to detect any reversible or irreversible contraindications to MSG, as suggested by Pignataro et al in 2008.[13]

7.2.1 Case History Collection

Detailed case history collection should focus on identification of any general and specific risk factors for MSG and/or sinonasal disease, including history of allergic rhinitis, previous nasal surgery or trauma, history of chronic or recurrent rhinosinusitis or nasal polyposis, the chronic use of nasal steroids or vasoconstrictors (which indicates a possible underlying sinonasal disease), previous treatment for head and neck malignancies, smoking (active or passive exposure), and the presence of any comorbidity known to impair mucociliary clearance (such as cystic fibrosis, Kartagener's syndrome and primary ciliary dyskinesia, use of ciliostatic drugs) or associated with sinonasal disease (such as asthma, chronic obstructive pulmonary disease, peripheral hypereosinophilia, and acetylsalicylic acid hypersensitivity). If anamnestic data identify any of these risk factors, the patient should undergo an ENT evaluation.[14] ▶ Fig. 7.1 is a data and history collection sheet that can be used by dentists and oral surgeons to evaluate if a given patient is a candidate for further ENT examination.

7.2.2 Imaging

Every MSG candidate should undergo appropriate radiological evaluation with the aim of visualizing not only the upper dental arch and the overlying maxillary sinus, but also the ostiomeatal complex (OMC). Therefore,

---

Date_____

PERSONAL AND DEMOGRAPHIC INFORMATION

Surname:_____ First name:_____

Gender: □ male   □ female   Telephone number:_____

Surgical planning:_____ Side: □ left   □ right

GENERAL INFORMATION

Smoking: □ no   □ yes
Diabetes: □ no   □ yes
Vasculopathy/Immune disease: □ no   □ yes
Specify:_____
Chronic drugs assumption: :   □ no   □ yes
Specify:_____
Allergy: □ no   □ yes
Specify:_____
ASA hypersensitivity: □ no   □ yes
Addiction to sniffing drugs: □ no   □ yes
Specify:_____
Pulmonary disease: □ no   □ yes   Specify: □ Asthma
                                                                       □ COPD
                                                                       □ Bronchiectasis

Other:_____
Congenital systemic disease: □ no   □ yes   Specify: □ Cystic fibrosis
                                                                       □ Primary ciliary dyskinesia
                                                                       □ Kartagener's disease
                                                                       □ Peripheral hypereosinophilia

                                                              Other:_____

Primary or secondary immune defect: □ no   □ yes
Specify:_____

SPECIFIC INFORMATION

Perceived nasal obstruction: □ no   □ yes
Recurrent or chronic nasal discharge: □ no   □ yes
Recurrent or chronic headache: □ no   □ yes
Specify:_____
Loss of smell :   □ no   □ yes
History of rhinosinusitis: □ no   □ yes
History of nasosinusal polyposis: □ no   □ yes

Fig. 7.1 History collection sheet. This brief survey is designed to help oral and maxillofacial surgeons evaluate candidates for maxillary sinus grafting. Patients who give any positive answers to these questions should undergo an ENT evaluation prior to maxillary sinus grafting. The sheet can be photocopied and reproduced, provided that the book and the authors are acknowledged. This tool may also allow specialists and researchers to collect data on MSG candidates in a standardized format.

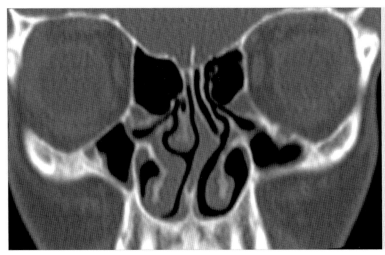

Fig. 7.2 Reversible contraindication to maxillary sinus grafting. A left septal deviation displacing the homolateral middle turbinate and closing the ostiomeatal complex in the presence of bilateral Haller cells is an easily manageable contraindication to MSG. After the septal deviation is corrected and the Haller cells opened, the MSG can be performed safely, allowing for successful implant placement.

preoperative radiological evaluation should include not only traditional orthopantomography, but also CT scans extending to the ethmoidal roof. Thanks to the rapid evolution of CT technology, cone-beam devices are widely available and allow for a reduced radiation dose, while maintaining good accuracy. While traditional CT scans represent a viable alternative for MSG candidates, DentaScans (or low-detail cone-beam CT limited to only the dental arch) do not provide sufficient data for patient evaluation. See Chapter 2 (p. 16) for further information on radiological evaluation of patients.

7.3 Reversible and Irreversible Contraindications

As we have already stated in the Introduction, the better the starting condition of the sinonasal complex, the lower the risk of complications after maxillary augmentation. Therefore, when we evaluate from an ENT point of view a potential candidate for MSG, we must bear in mind two questions: (1) Are there conditions that contraindicate MSG? and (2) Can I solve these unfavorable conditions or are they irreversible?

For example, if a candidate for MSG presents with a septal deviation obstructing the OMC on the homolateral side to the planned augmentation, with middle turbinate lateralization, there is a risk of insufficient ventilation and clearance after the grafting procedure. This situation may lead to stasis of sinusal secretions and development of a sinus infection. In these patients, a simple surgical procedure may guarantee ostium patency in the early postaugmentation period, ensuring a safe MSG. This initial, potentially unfavorable condition is therefore *reversible* (▶ Fig. 7.2). In contrast, if a candidate for MSG presents with cystic fibrosis, we cannot expect any significant improvement in his or her sinonasal condition, despite the best medical and surgical care we can provide.

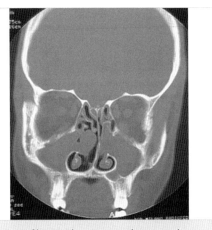

Fig. 7.3 Cystic fibrosis. The secretory alterations characterizing patients with cystic fibrosis radically impair the mucociliary drainage of the sinonasal complex. In this CT scan we can appreciate the complete opacification of both maxillary sinuses with progressive resorption of the uncinate process, which is pathognomonic of this condition. In this patient, the correct ostiomeatal complex drainage cannot be restored, either surgically or medically.

This contraindication is therefore, at present, *irreversible* (▶ Fig. 7.3).

Bearing in mind these two simple but important questions, we will provide a complete list of sinonasal contraindications to MSG, distinguishing between reversible and irreversible contraindications.

7.3.1 Reversible Contraindications

Among ENT contraindications to MSG, the reversible ones are by far the most frequent, and these should be corrected in order to completely restore maxillary sinus drainage and ventilation by means of the most appropriate medical and/or surgical approach. Many are electively amenable to functional endoscopic sinus surgery, which is currently the mainstay minimally invasive option for surgical treatment of most sinonasal disease.

Reversible ENT contraindications to MSG are[13,15]:

- Any anatomo-structural situation significantly impairing the patency of the OMC and potentially leading to reduced sinusal drainage and ventilation, with or without preoperative maxillary sinusitis. They include: conspicuous septal deviation impairing the middle meatus; large paradoxical bending of the middle turbinate; concha bullosa; hypertrophy of the agger nasi; Haller cell

or pneumatization of the uncinate process reducing OMC patency; and postsurgical or posttraumatic synechiae of the OMC (▶ Fig. 7.4). It is extremely important to remember that these findings do not represent a contraindication per se: they should be addressed only when they represent an obstacle to ventilation and drainage of the OMC. Small anomalies not affecting OMC patency or anomalies on the opposite side to the grafting should not be addressed surgically on a purely implant-related basis.

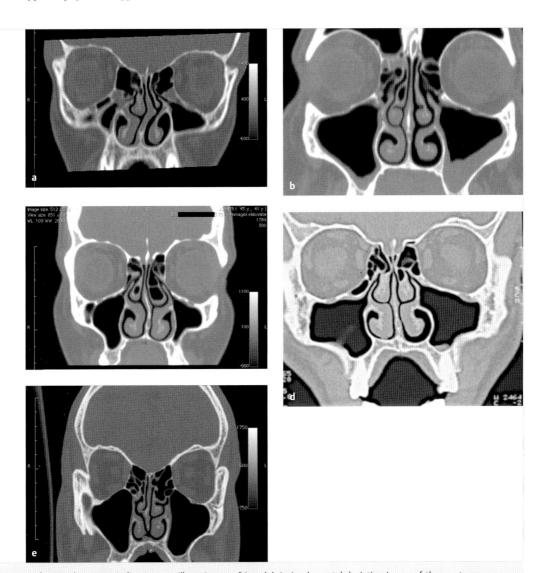

Fig. 7.4 Anatomical anomalies contraindicating maxillary sinus grafting. **(a)** A simple septal deviation is one of the most common findings in patients undergoing ENT evaluation before MSG. In this patient the deviation partially obstructs the left ostiomeatal complex. Signs of dysventilation and mucosal hyperplasia can be identified in the ethmoidal cells bilaterally. **(b)** Another common anomaly is the paradoxical bending of the middle nasal concha: the convexity of the turbinate faces the ostiomeatal complex, which is therefore narrowed. **(c)** Similarly, a concha bullosa (i.e., a middle nasal concha containing an air chamber) significantly reduces OMC patency. **(d)** Haller cells, which are extraethmoidal air cells lying inferiorly to the orbit, significantly reduce the drainage area of the maxillary sinus owing to their close proximity to the natural ostium of the sinus. **(e)** Small synechiae (i.e., bridges of scar tissue connecting anatomical structures that are normally independent) can form following nasal surgery or trauma or—exceptionally—may have a congenital origin.

- Any inflammatory or infectious (related to viral, bacterial, or fungal etiology) sinusal process. The former includes: allergic rhinosinusitis and sinonasal polyposis groups I to IV according to Stammberger's classification (group I, antrochoanal polyps, see ▶ Fig. 7.5; group II, isolated large polyps; group III, polyps associated with chronic rhinosinusitis, noneosinophil-dominated and not related to hyperreactive airway; group IV, polyps associated with chronic rhinosinusitis, eosinophil dominated)[16] (▶ Fig. 7.6). Infectious processes include: acute viral or bacterial rhinosinusitis (▶ Fig. 7.7); fungus ball (noninvasive fungal rhinosinusitis) (▶ Fig. 7.8); recurrent and chronic rhinosinusitis, possibly caused by one of the aforementioned anatomical situations impairing maxillary drainage (▶ Fig. 7.9).
- Antral foreign bodies (such as displaced dental implants or any other migrated prosthetic material) with or without reactive maxillary sinus involvement (▶ Fig. 7.10).
- Oroantral fistulae (▶ Fig. 7.11).
- Benign sinonasal neoplasms/malformations and space-occupying inflammatory lesions that reduce the patency of the maxillary drainage pathway. These include: large mucous cysts (▶ Fig. 7.12); cholesterinic granulomas; juvenile angiofibroma extending to the middle meatus; and inverted papillomas of the nose and ethmoid (▶ Fig. 7.13). From a purely implant-related point of view, these conditions represent a contraindication to MSG only if homolateral to the side of the skull where the grafting is planned. Non implant-related considerations concerning the opportunity to treat these conditions are well beyond the scope of this book.
- All these conditions can be surgically treated prior to or in association with MSG, thus achieving both OMC rehabilitation and restoration of an effective mucociliary clearance system, resulting in a complete recovery of sinonasal homeostasis.

7.3.2 Irreversible Contraindications

Irreversible ENT contraindications to MSG include all the conditions considered to permanently alter maxillary sinus homeostasis by irreversibly interfering with at least one of the following: the patency of the anatomical drainage pathway, the adequate synthesis and composition of mucous secretions, and the efficacy of the epithelial ciliary movement.

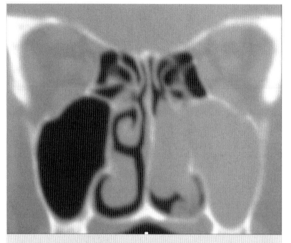

Fig. 7.5 Solitary unilateral polyps protruding from the maxillary sinus ostium are commonly called antrochoanal polyps. They may recur due to failure to remove their stalk, usually located in the lower part of the maxillary sinus.

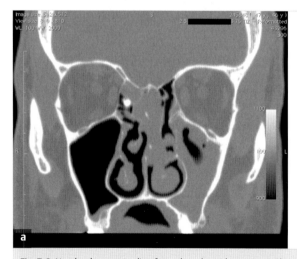
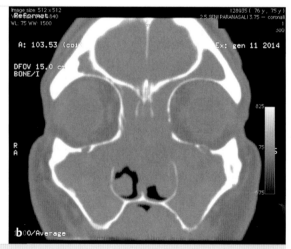

Fig. 7.6 Nasal polyps protruding from the ethmoid can impair the nasal fossa ventilation to a varying extent, from (a) mild forms to (b) massive obliterating forms. Nasal polyps have a definite tendency to recur, which is significantly higher in massive forms and in patients presenting with asthma and aspirin intolerance.

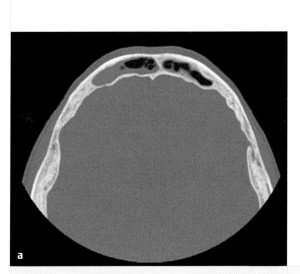
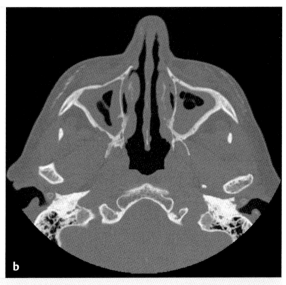

Fig. 7.7 Acute rhinosinusitis. In this patient, suffering from acute bacterial pansinusitis, the acute inflammatory condition is suggested by the air–fluid levels and bubbles that can be identified both in (a) the frontal sinuses and (b) the maxillary sinus.

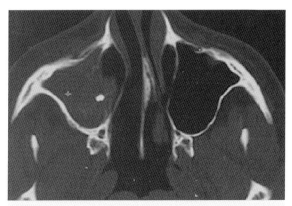

Fig. 7.8 Maxillary fungus ball. These chronic inflammatory fungal conditions have a noninvasive extramucosal localization. As stated in Chapter 6 (p. 84), these infections have a distinctive ironlike density in CT scans, often accompanied by a mild bone thickening.

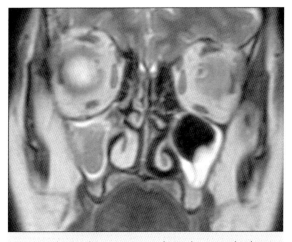

Fig. 7.9 Chronic rhinosinusitis. Head MRI showing right chronic rhinosinusitis. The MR signals identify both the reactive mucosal hyperplasia and the fluid obliterating the whole right maxillary sinus. The chronic inflammatory condition also induced a reactive hyperplasia of the left maxillary sinus, which was not followed by fluid accumulation.

These conditions are frequently intrinsic features of underlying systemic pathologies associated with chronic sinusal diseases. Under such circumstances, the maxillary sinusal drainage and/or the mucociliary clearance are permanently impaired, with a consequent decrease in antral oxygen concentration. This leads to epithelial dysfunction, which predisposes to infection and edema of the OMC, thus further impairing maxillary drainage and ventilation.

As previously mentioned, no data are currently available regarding the presumed negative outcome of MSG in such patients, but one may speculate that when sinusal compliance is greatly reduced, the risk of development of

sinus-related complications after MSG would not be negligible. Therefore, we suggest avoiding MSG in patients with the following clinical conditions[13,15]:
• Any anatomo-structural situation significantly and permanently impairing the patency of the OMC or the physiological status of the maxillary mucosa that is not suitable for complete correction. These include: large postsurgical, posttraumatic, or radiation-induced sequelae involving the OMC or Schneider's membrane (▶ Fig. 7.14).

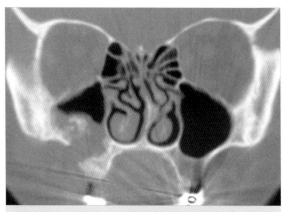

Fig. 7.10 Chronic rhinosinusitis following infection and displacement of maxillary sinus grafting material into the maxillary sinus. Note both the free-floating calcifications in the sinus (autologous bony particles) and the oroantral communication resulting from the maxillary sinus grafting procedure and the subsequent infection.

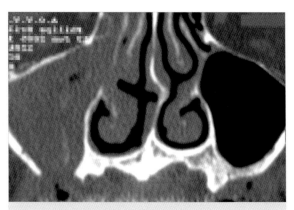

Fig. 7.11 Oroantral fistula. This patient is suffering from chronic right maxillary sinusitis after a maxillary sinus grafting procedure. The grafting material (autologous bone chips) can be observed floating toward the maxillary ostium, while a wide oroantral fistula, resulting from the maxillary grafting procedure, is visible in the lower part of the maxillary sinus.

- Any inflammatory or infectious sinusal process, including recurrent or chronic rhinosinusitis with or without nasal polyps, that cannot be solved by medical and/or surgical treatments because it is associated with systemic disease. These include: congenital disorders with impaired mucociliary clearance (e.g., cystic fibrosis, Kartagener's syndrome, Young's syndrome); Samter's triad (defined by acetylsalicylic acid hypersensitivity, sinonasal polyps, and asthma); immune defects (e.g., congenital and acquired immune disorders).
- Specific systemic granulomatosis diseases with sinonasal involvement, including sarcoidosis and Wegener's granulomatosis.
- Large benign and malignant sinonasal neoplasms directly affecting the maxillary sinus, the OMC, or nearby anatomical structures that seriously impair maxillary sinus homeostasis both before and after their treatment. Benign neoplasms include: excessively large inverted papillomas that require extensive and destructive surgery, with scarring and pathological alterations of drainage and anatomy; and fibro-osseous lesions of the ethmoid–maxillary complex. Malignant neoplasms include: primary malignant lesions originating from the epithelium, neuroectoderm, bone, soft tissue, dental tissue, and lymphatic system, and metastases (▶ Fig. 7.15).

7.4 Treatment of Reversible Contraindications

As we have already stated, reversible contraindications represent the most frequent scenario the oral surgeon and the ENT specialist have to face in planning MSG.

Such reversible contraindications can be resolved with adequate medical or surgical therapy that leads to normal maxillary sinus ventilation and drainage, thereby favoring uneventful graft integration. See also ▶ Table 7.1 for a quick reference to treatment choices. Medical and surgical management will be described in detail for each contraindication later in this chapter; other information on the surgical management of sinonasal diseases has already been covered in Chapter 6 (p. 84).

In 2008, we published a flow chart for the integrated management of candidates for MSG, including the treatment of reversible contraindications, and this should still be considered valid (▶ Fig. 7.16).

The most debated issue regarding reversible contraindications is not how to treat them (there is a general consensus among the ENT community about the medical and/or surgical gold standard of treatment for these pathoses or anatomical abnormalities), but what time interval should be adopted between the resolution of the contraindication and MSG. After medical treatment and, more significantly, after surgical treatment, the sinonasal mucosa invariably needs adequate healing time to allow swelling to reduce sufficiently and an efficient mucociliary transport to be restored. Unfortunately, there are no retrospective or prospective studies on this "safety time window" between treatment and grafting. However, as a 3- to 6-month period between treatment and grafting[17] seems to be an acceptable compromise between safety and early prosthetic rehabilitation, only strict cooperation between the ENT surgeon and the surgeon in charge of the MSG procedure can ensure successful grafting.[18]

An endoscopic examination of sinonasal healing after treating a reversible complication allows the otolaryngologist to predict the safety of maxillary grafting. Reports of diffuse crusting, excessive mucosal

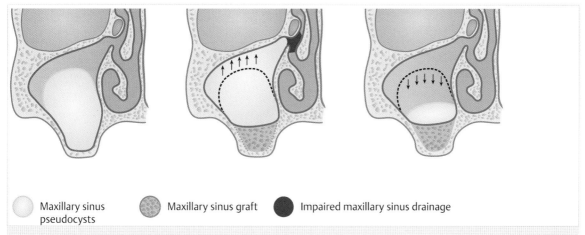

○ Maxillary sinus   ◔ Maxillary sinus graft   ● Impaired maxillary sinus drainage
pseudocysts

Fig. 7.12 Maxillary sinus cysts. Mucous retention cysts of the maxillary sinus do not normally impair mucociliary clearance and sinusal drainage. Nevertheless, when maxillary sinus grafting is performed, the cyst is elevated and may impact on the natural ostium, thus blocking the mucosal drainage and possibly causing inflammatory or infective conditions. If the cyst is deflated through an oral access or removed through an endoscopic antrostomy, the sinus floor can be elevated safely.

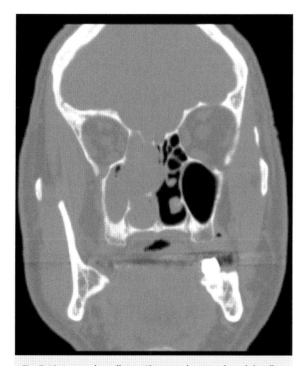

Fig. 7.13 Inverted papilloma. These are benign, though locally invasive, neoplasms of the maxillary sinus or ethmoidal cells. They can be completely removed, sparing most of the mucosa of the sinonasal cavity and thus not endangering its homeostasis. The effective sparing of the mucosa, and the chances of performing a maxillary sinus grafting after removal of the neoplasm, obviously depend on the size and position of the papilloma.

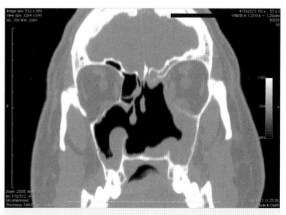

Fig. 7.14 Postoperative CT scan after wide endoscopic resection of a malignant tumor (intestinal-type adenocarcinoma). Most bone walls and most of the mucosal lining are missing. Though the patient is not suffering from an inflammatory condition, and despite the successful tumor resection, the mucociliary clearance is completely disrupted, favoring crusting and continuous scarring.

swelling endangering the patency of the antrostomy, or, even worse, overabundant secretion, suggest the grafting procedure should be postponed. On the other hand, a healthy mucosa with patent nasal cavities, sinusal ostia,

and sinusal cavities provides a green light for maxillary sinus augmentation, allowing the surgeon to avoid further unhelpful and potentially confusing imaging studies. For example, mucosal hypertrophy, a frequent finding during radiological examination of the maxillary sinus, does not represent a sign of inflammation, although it is often misinterpreted by radiologists. Mucosal hypertrophy is often a permanent sequela of surgery. It causes a slight reduction in the volume of the maxillary sinus without altering its physiology.

However, if we take into account the safety time proposed by this protocol (3–6 months between treatment of the contraindication and grafting) and we sum it with:

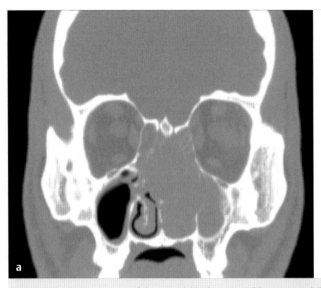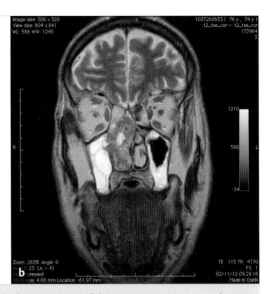

Fig. 7.15 Malignant tumors of the nose. **(a)** Esthesioneuroblastomas and **(b)** adenocarcinomas of the nose require extensive endoscopic surgery in order to protect the patient from recurrences. In order to maximize the oncological chances of success, the common functional features of endoscopic sinus surgery are jeopardized: the mucosal lining is stripped from wide peritumoral areas and the bone walls are opened in order to grant access and facilitate radical resection.

Table 7.1 Treatment choices for reversible contraindications

Suggested treatment	Type of contraindication	Minimum suggested treatment-to-grafting interval	Additional imaging	Pregrafting endoscopy to confirm healing
Medical treatment with delayed maxillary sinus grafting	Acute viral or bacterial sinusitis, common cold, influenza	1 month	No	Yes
Surgical treatment with delayed maxillary sinus grafting	CRS with polyps, fungus ball, recurrent sinusitis with significant chronic mucosal edema, foreign body sinusitis, oroantral fistula	3 months	No	Yes
	Locally invasive benign neoplasms (juvenile angiofibroma, inverted papilloma)	6 months	Yes (MRI)	Yes
Surgical treatment with simultaneous maxillary sinus grafting	Septal deviation, paradoxical bending of the middle turbinate, concha bullosa, hypertrophy of the agger nasi, Haller cell or pneumatization of the uncinate process, postsurgical or posttraumatic synechiae, antral foreign body without inflammation, large mucous cysts, choanal polyps, cholesterinic granulomas, recurrent sinusitis with minimal mucosal alterations	None	Not applicable	Not applicable

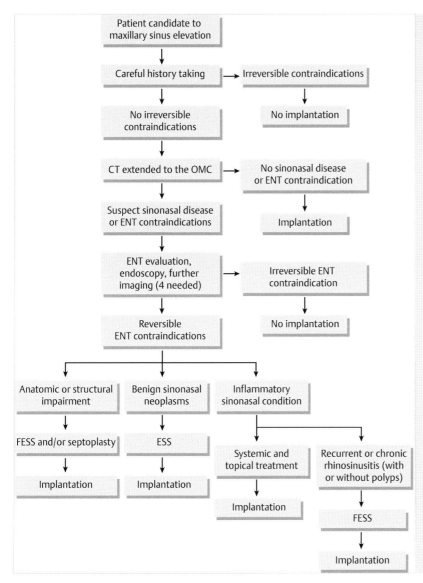

Fig. 7.16 Flow chart for the integrated management of candidates for maxillary sinus grafting, including the treatment of reversible contraindications. CT, computed tomography; ESS, endoscopic sinus surgery; FESS, functional endoscopic sinus surgery; OMC, ostiomeatal complex.

(1) the 6- to 9-month period generally requested for maxillary graft integration; (2) the 2- to 3-month period needed for implant integration; and (3) the prosthetic restoration times, we come up with long rehabilitation times.

In order to reduce treatment times, Felisati et al[19] proposed a combined procedure in 2010, in which both the treatment of the sinonasal contraindication and the MSG procedure are performed at the same time.

We can therefore classify reversible ENT contraindications to MSG according to the treatment required: medical treatment with delayed MSG, surgical treatment with delayed MSG, and surgical treatment with simultaneous MSG (▶ Table 7.1).

7.4.1 Medical Treatment of Reversible Contraindications

Clinical evidence of acute rhinosinusitis (ARS), whether viral or bacterial, and signs or symptoms of viral infection of the upper respiratory tract are temporary contraindications to MSG, owing to the higher risk of graft infection.

Bacterial and viral rhinosinusitis are very often difficult to distinguish, and ENT specialist referral should be considered only for patients whose condition is severe or not improving. Complete ARS management is well beyond the scope of this book and the EPOS document from the European Rhinological Society[20] provides a free and complete guide to ENT specialists and nonspecialists. As a

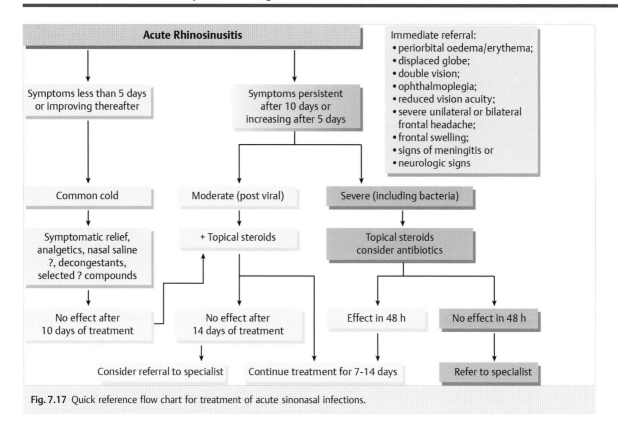

Fig. 7.17 Quick reference flow chart for treatment of acute sinonasal infections.

quick reference to treatment and management, please see ▶ Fig. 7.17. Antibiotics should be reserved for patients whose condition is severe or not improving; oral amoxicillin and clavulanate (1 g, 3 times per day) is a common and useful choice, while oral levofloxacin (500 mg per day) or oral clarithromycin (500 mg, 2 times per day) is the medication of choice in patients with a history of adverse drug reactions with β-lactam drugs. Symptomatic topical treatments (decongestants and saline irrigations) and systemic drugs (analgesics) can be employed, while steroid use, both topical and systemic, is encouraged in moderate or severe patients for symptom relief.

After correct treatment of the infection, a 30-day waiting period is advisable to obtain adequate OMC patency and mucosal trophism. This period is generally enough to minimize the chance of a relapse. No further imaging examinations are required to sanction the MSG, although an endoscopic examination may prove useful to ensure healing and reassure the patient.

7.4.2 Surgical Treatment with Delayed Maxillary Sinus Grafting

One of the most common contraindications amenable to surgical treatment is chronic rhinosinusitis (CRS). CRS, with or without polyps, is one of the most complex and

debated subjects in otorhinolaryngology and countless articles and books continue to expand the debate every month.

The surgical mainstay for treating these conditions is functional endoscopic sinus surgery (FESS). With FESS, the surgeon is able to restore adequate sinonasal drainage and ventilation by enlarging the sinusal ostia and opening the ethmoidal cells, with a minimally invasive approach, low patient discomfort, and a more than acceptable complication rate. When treating a patient with CRS for implant-related purposes, the goals remain the same as for other patients, but with keener attention to the maxillary sinus. The treatment should be addressed to all involved cavities, in order to drain infective foci and restore ventilation, while healthy sinuses should be left untreated. Care should be taken not to induce excessive scarring, and it is essential to simultaneously treat any anatomical anomaly, such as septal deviation, conchae bullosa, etc., that could endanger the drainage. After successful healing of the mucosa (3 months are generally needed), the MSG procedure can be performed.

Although recurrences of CRS without polyps are quite frequent, even after a properly conducted procedure, the sinus graft is given enough time to integrate into the subsinusal space created by maxillary sinus elevation, thanks to the restoration of physiological mucosal drainage and ventilation of the sinus. Medical therapy consisting of intranasal steroids may be useful to reduce postoperative edema and recurrences.

Other reversible contraindications, such as fungus balls, foreign body sinusitis, oroantral fistulae, and sinonasal complications of dental disease and treatment (SCDDT) may interfere with a safe MSG and must be resolved prior to sinus grafting according to the SCDDT standard protocols already described in Chapter 6 (p. 84).[18]

Although not as frequent as CRS, other reversible pathoses, such as locally invasive benign neoplasms, often require complex surgical endoscopic procedures. It is beyond the scope of this textbook to analyze the surgical details, but it is nevertheless worth noting that the treatment of these neoplasms is mainly endoscopic, and radical resection of the tumor is the main goal of the surgical procedure. On the other hand, the ENT specialist should bear in mind that sparing most of the nasal structures is essential for safe MSG: excessively destructive procedures such as extremely large maxillectomies or septal ablations induce air vortices, crusting, and pooling of secretions, which may potentially endanger the MSG procedure. If too much of the mucoperiosteal lining of the maxillary sinus is removed, Schneider's membrane will be replaced by thick scar tissue covering the maxillary sinus. This new lining, despite its thickness, is often fragile and difficult to elevate during MSG. In these patients, CT and MR imaging, in addition to endoscopic examination, are mandatory to confirm the absence of local recurrences before planning an MSG procedure.

7.4.3 Surgical Treatment with Simultaneous Maxillary Sinus Grafting

A staged surgical approach on one hand allows an MSG procedure to be performed on an already healed maxillary sinus, but on the other hand prolongs rehabilitation times as described at the beginning of Section 7.4 (p. 134). The combined procedure proposed by Felisati et al in 2010,[19] in which treatment of the sinonasal contraindication and the MSG procedure are performed simultaneously, reduces treatment times considerably. However, it should be noted that this approach is limited to noninfective sinonasal conditions, because of the nonnegligible risk of contaminating the graft. Conversely, in patients with unexpected intraoperative findings of ongoing infection (undiagnosed fungus balls, purulent antral or ethmoidal secretions), the endoscopic surgery must be performed, but MSG should be postponed for at least 3 months.

Clinical conditions that can be treated with a combined approach include anatomical anomalies such as

posttraumatic synechiae, paradoxical bending of the middle turbinate, concha bullosa, hypertrophy of the agger nasi, Haller cells, and pneumatization of the uncinate process, as well as minor maxillary neoformations such as choanal polyps, cholesterinic granulomas, and mucous cysts. It must be remembered that these conditions should be treated only when they create a significant obstacle to the OMC on the side(s) scheduled for grafting.

This combined treatment requires the collaboration of an ENT surgeon and an oral/maxillofacial surgeon. The procedure involves two surgical steps. The first step is the nasal procedure, most often carried out endoscopically, which aims to eliminate the pathological condition that is a contraindication to the MSG procedure; the second step is the oral procedure, with the creation of the maxillary bony window and insertion of the graft under Schneider's membrane. Significant septal deviations can be treated either endoscopically (particularly in patients with localized posterior deviations or septal spurs) or with the classic technique proposed by Cottle,[21] which employs nasal specula and a headlight to provide a view of the nasal cavity. It is nevertheless advisable to perform an endoscopic inspection of the sinonasal complex even after carrying out a traditional septoplasty, owing to the significant role played by the OMC in a successful grafting. Postsurgical or posttraumatic synechiae are quickly addressed endoscopically with laser, lancet, or scissors. The procedure is minimally invasive and can also be carried out under local anesthesia, if the synechiae are easy to address.

Patients suffering from recurrent sinusitis with minimal mucosal alterations are often safely amenable to combined treatment. These patients generally have no infective reservoirs and show minimal mucosal thickening due to local airflow disturbances (anatomical anomalies are commonplace in these patients). Opening of the sinusal ostia and ethmoidal cells can therefore be carried out endoscopically at the time of MSG, thereby reducing the risk of infection and guaranteeing good maxillary sinus drainage. These patients should therefore undergo limited FESS procedures, with the same methods and instruments used in patients suffering from more extensive CRS.

Other anatomical anomalies such as concha bullosa, hypertrophy of the agger nasi, Haller cells, and pneumatization of the uncinate process, as well as minor maxillary neoformations such as choanal polyps and cholesterinic granulomas, can easily be treated with an endoscopic approach at the same time as MSG. See Chapter 6 (p. 84) for details.

Other benign lesions that may block the natural ostium after raising the maxillary sinus floor are large mucous cysts. These are found in approximately 7% of the adult population and represent about 90% of all the cystic lesions that can affect the paranasal sinuses.

Development of the lesion causes liquid accumulation between the epithelial and the periosteal layers of Schneider's membrane, leading to a natural separation of the two anatomical layers. These cysts are primarily located over the sinus floor, and in most patients are totally asymptomatic.[22] Their detection is usually fortuitous and consequent to routine radiographic assessments that reveal a typical well-defined "dome-shaped" radiopaque lesion. When patients are scheduled for sinus elevation, the presence of a small cyst arising from the sinus floor hardly represents a significant contraindication to the procedure, as obstruction of the ostium is unlikely to occur.[23–25] In contrast, large cysts (occupying at least one-third of the sinus volume) may interfere with membrane mobilization, increase the risk of iatrogenic membrane perforation, and promote maxillary ostium obstruction. Membrane perforation may be followed by contamination of the grafting material and/or its dispersion into the maxillary sinus, potentially leading to inflammatory foreign body reactions and/or sinus infections. Ostium obstruction after completion of the grafting procedure may potentially lead to mucus accumulation within the maxillary sinus, loss of sinus ventilation, and sinus infection.[13,19] Therefore, it may be advisable to remove large cysts prior to or during a sinus grafting procedure.

Cysts can be removed either endoscopically after a surgical antrostomy, or through an intraoral approach. The latter can be performed with the creation of a bony window pedicled to Schneider's membrane, as described in Chapter 6 (p.84), or via a microaccess through the anterolateral wall of the sinus. In the latter case, the anterolateral wall of the maxillary sinus requiring grafting is exposed and a bony window is outlined to perform a standard sinus floor elevation procedure, as described in Chapter 6 (p.84). Prior to membrane mobilization and sinus grafting, an additional small circular bony access (less than 5 mm in diameter) is made above the cranial margin of the sinus lift osteotomy. An intentional perforation of the membrane through the additional bony access allows an approach to the underlying cystic lesion. Preliminary suction of the cystic liquid is performed to significantly reduce the cyst volume and simplify its removal. As the ciliated epithelium and the periosteum of Schneider's membrane have been naturally separated into two different layers by the hydrostatic pressure generated by the endocystic liquid, it is relatively easy to remove the collapsed cystic walls through the small accessory bony access by means of a fine surgical suction tip and tissue pliers. The integrity of the periosteal layer of Schneider's membrane remaining over the sinus elevation site can be checked through the standard osteotomy created for sinus grafting. The surgical procedure is then completed, following the well-known steps of the traditional sinus grafting protocol (▶ Fig. 7.18).

It is worth noting that if an antrostomy has been performed during the combined procedure, it will be possible for the ENT surgeon to endoscopically follow the sinus grafting procedure and to check the integrity of Schneider's membrane. If a perforation occurs, it can be promptly identified and the oral surgeon will take care of closing it, either by further unfolding the membrane or using a resorbable barrier, as described in Chapter 6 (p.84), to avoid penetration of the grafting material into the sinus cavity (see ▶ Fig. 3.17, ▶ Fig. 3.19).

Key Points

- Maxillary sinus grafting is a safe procedure, as long as the maxillary sinus is healthy, the ostiomeatal complex patent, and the secretion drainage efficient.
- Conditions that reduce or block the mucosal drainage from the maxillary sinus represent contraindications to the grafting procedure.
- Patients with known or suspected sinonasal disorders should undergo ENT evaluation and adequate imaging prior to grafting.
- The candidate for maxillary sinus grafting may suffer from either reversible or irreversible contraindications.
- According to the specific type of reversible contraindication, treatment can be medical or surgical and, in some patients, can even be combined with the maxillary sinus grafting procedure.
- Patients with severe sinonasal inflammatory conditions should be addressed with endoscopic sinus surgery, irrespective of the indication for maxillary sinus grafting. The sinus should be grafted after at least 4 months from the endoscopic procedure. On the other hand, patients with mild chronic sinonasal conditions should undergo endoscopic sinus surgery to allow for maxillary sinus grafting. Endoscopic sinus surgery and maxillary grafting can also be performed in the same surgical setting. Lastly, significant OMC anatomical alteration without signs of sinonasal inflammation should undergo endoscopic surgical correction in order to minimize the chance of graft failure. Surgical treatment of OMC anomalies and grafting can also be performed in the same surgical setting.

7.5 Clinical Cases

7.5.1 Case 1

The patient is a 53-year-old man, a candidate for bilateral MSG for prosthetic purposes. During history-taking he reported two or three episodes per year of recurring headache with purulent discharge and occasionally fever over the last 5 years. The patient was therefore referred to an ENT specialist, who asked for a CT scan of the head. The case is shown in ▶ Fig. 7.19. See also ▶Video 7.1.

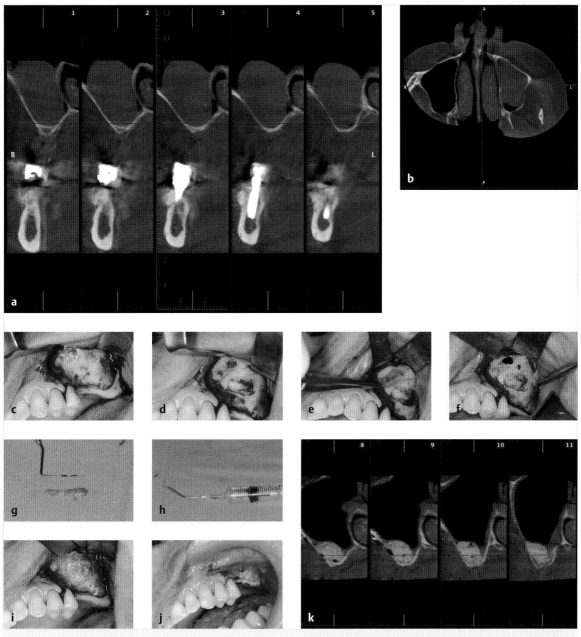

Fig. 7.18 (a,b) Mucous cyst of the left maxillary sinus in a patient who is a candidate for sinus grafting (MSG), which may interfere with ostium patency at the end of the MSG procedure. **(c)** Elevation of an intraoral flap. **(d)** Creation of the bony window for the MSG procedure and the microaccess to remove the cyst. **(e–h)** Removal of the cyst through the microaccess. **(i,j)** Sinus grafting and closure of the flap. **(k)** CT scan at the end of the procedure: the sinus graft is clearly visible and the cyst has disappeared.

7.5.2 Case 2

The patient is a 65-year-old man with a history of nasal breathing disorders without sinusitis, dating back to his thirties. The patient had already been diagnosed with a right posttraumatic septal deviation, but had refused surgery, many years previously. The patient was a candidate for a bilateral maxillary sinus elevation and was therefore referred to an ENT specialist due to his known rhinological comorbidities. The ENT specialist asked for a cone-beam CT scan of the head, which the patient had not previously undergone. The case is shown in ▶ Fig. 7.20. See also ▶ Video 7.2.

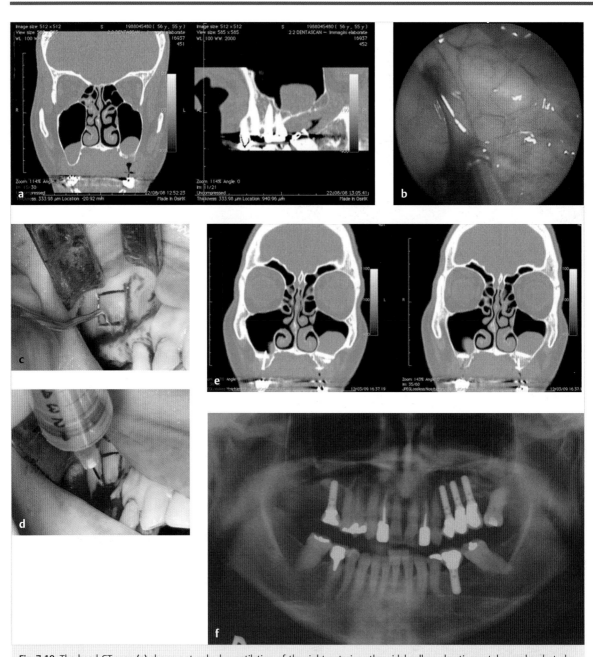

Fig. 7.19 The head CT scan (**a**) shows not only dysventilation of the right anterior ethmoidal cells and ostiomeatal complex, but also bilateral maxillary sinus cysts. The left ostiomeatal complex is relatively patent and shows no dysventilation signs. Note also the reduced, insufficient, bone height in the coronal images (right). The patient was therefore selected as a candidate for a combined endoscopic endonasal and oral procedure. The endonasal procedure was aimed at enhancing the maxillary sinus drainage through a wide antrostomy (**b**), which also allowed direct vision of the cyst, and medializing the right middle turbinate in order to widen the right ostiomeatal complex. In the same surgical setting a bone window was created in the lower part of the maxillary bone (**c**), not only for grafting purposes but also to allow deflating the cyst with a simple syringe (**d**). With this maneuver, the sinus was protected from the risks of raising the cyst, without excessive trauma or perforation of Schneider's membrane. The left maxillary cyst and sinus were not addressed surgically, as there were no signs of dysventilation or blockade of the ostiomeatal complex. At 3-month radiographic follow-up (**e**), the head CT scan shows successful integration of the graft in both maxillary sinuses, without signs of infection or inflammation. The mild ethmoidal mucosal hyperplasia shown in the preoperative CT scan has been successfully treated. Note also the wide right surgical antrostomy allowing for proper drainage. The right maxillary cyst did not recur. A 6-month postoperative orthopantomography (**f**) shows the complete prosthetic rehabilitation of the patient without signs of infection.

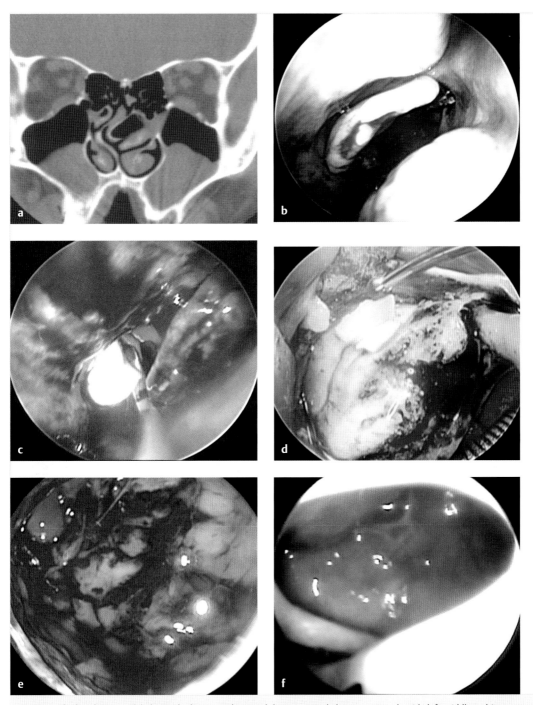

Fig. 7.20 The head CT scan **(a)** shows the known right septal deviation, and also an extremely wide left middle turbinate concha bullosa. The left ostiomeatal complex was therefore almost completely closed and dysventilation signs are shown on the scan. The CT scan also showed bilateral maxillary sinus cysts, which should be considered another reversible contraindication to maxillary sinus grafting. On explaining to the patient the risks his rhinological condition posed to future maxillary sinus grafting, he gave his consent to a combined endoscopic endonasal and oral procedure. The patient therefore underwent in the same surgical setting a left middle conchoplasty **(b)**, removing the lateral half of the concha and restoring ostiomeatal complex patency, and a traditional septoplasty. The left cysts were excised through a wide antrostomy **(c)**, thus freeing the sinus from potential obstruction upon elevation. A sinus lift was then performed through a classic oral access **(d)**. The combined procedure allowed for endoscopic control of the integrity of Schneider's membrane through the antrostomy **(e)**. At 6-month follow-up the patient had healed completely and the graft was integrated without signs, as the endoscopic control confirmed **(f)**. There was a significant improvement in his quality of life, due to the resolution of his nasal breathing difficulties.

References

[1] Moreno Vazquez JC, Gonzalez de Rivera AS, Gil HS, Mifsut RS. Complication rate in 200 consecutive sinus lift procedures: guidelines for prevention and treatment. J Oral Maxillofac Surg 2014; 72: 892–901

[2] Zimbler MS, Lebowitz RA, Glickman R, Brecht LE, Jacobs JB. Antral augmentation, osseointegration, and sinusitis: the otolaryngologist's perspective. Am J Rhinol 1998; 12: 311–316

[3] Jensen J, Reiche-Fischel O, Sindet-Pedersen S. Autogenous mandibular bone grafts for malar augmentation. J Oral Maxillofac Surg 1995; 53: 88–90

[4] Raghoebar GM, Vissink A, Reintsema H, Batenburg RH. Bone grafting of the floor of the maxillary sinus for the placement of endosseous implants. Br J Oral Maxillofac Surg 1997; 35: 119–125

[5] Timmenga NM, Raghoebar GM, Liem RS, van Weissenbruch R, Manson WL, Vissink A. Effects of maxillary sinus floor elevation surgery on maxillary sinus physiology. Eur J Oral Sci 2003; 111: 189–197

[6] Timmenga NM, Raghoebar GM, van Weissenbruch R, Vissink A. Maxillary sinus floor elevation surgery. A clinical, radiographic and endoscopic evaluation. Clin Oral Implants Res 2003; 14: 322–328

[7] Zinner ID, Small SA. Sinus-lift graft: using the maxillary sinuses to support implants. J Am Dent Assoc 1996; 127: 51–57

[8] Barone A, Santini S, Sbordone L, Crespi R, Covani U. A clinical study of the outcomes and complications associated with maxillary sinus augmentation. Int J Oral Maxillofac Implants 2006; 21: 81–85

[9] Bhattacharyya N. Bilateral chronic maxillary sinusitis after the sinus-lift procedure. Am J Otolaryngol 1999; 20: 133–135

[10] Ewers R. Maxilla sinus grafting with marine algae derived bone forming material: a clinical report of long-term results. J Oral Maxillofac Surg 2005; 63: 1712–1723

[11] Regev E, Smith RA, Perrott DH, Pogrel MA. Maxillary sinus complications related to endosseous implants. Int J Oral Maxillofac Implants 1995; 10: 451–461

[12] Timmenga NM, Raghoebar GM, Boering G, van Weissenbruch R. Maxillary sinus function after sinus lifts for the insertion of dental implants. J Oral Maxillofac Surg 1997; 55: 936–939, discussion 940

[13] Pignataro L, Mantovani M, Torretta S, Felisati G, Sambataro G. ENT assessment in the integrated management of candidate for (maxillary) sinus lift. Acta Otorhinolaryngol Ital 2008; 28: 110–119

[14] Cote MT, Segelnick SL, Rastogi A, Schoor R. New York state ear, nose, and throat specialists' views on pre-sinus lift referral. J Periodontol 2011; 82: 227–233

[15] Torretta S, Mantovani M, Testori T, Cappadona M, Pignataro L. Importance of ENT assessment in stratifying candidates for sinus floor elevation: a prospective clinical study. Clin Oral Implants Res 2013; 24 Suppl A100: 57–62

[16] Stammberger H. Surgical treatment of nasal polyps: past, present, and future. Allergy 1999; 54 Suppl 53: 7–11

[17] Colletti G, Felisati G, Biglioli F, Tintinelli R, Valassina D. Maxillary reconstruction and placement of dental implants after treatment of a maxillary sinus fungus ball. Int J Oral Maxillofac Implants 2010; 25: 1041–1044

[18] Felisati G, Saibene AM, Pipolo C, Mandelli F, Testori T. Implantology and otorhinolaryngology team-up to solve a complicated case. Implant Dent 2014; 23: 617–621

[19] Felisati G, Borloni R, Chiapasco M, Lozza P, Casentini P, Pipolo C. Maxillary sinus elevation in conjunction with transnasal endoscopic treatment of rhino-sinusal pathoses: preliminary results on 10 consecutively treated patients. Acta Otorhinolaryngol Ital 2010; 30: 289–293

[20] Fokkens WJ, Lund VJ, Mullol J et al. EPOS 2012: European position paper on rhinosinusitis and nasal polyps 2012. A summary for otorhinolaryngologists. Rhinology 2012; 50: 1–12

[21] Cottle MH, Loring RM. Surgery of the nasal septum; new operative procedures and indications. Ann Otol Rhinol Laryngol 1948; 57: 705–713

[22] Albu S. Symptomatic maxillary sinus retention cysts: should they be removed? Laryngoscope 2010; 120: 1904–1909

[23] Mardinger O, Manor I, Mijiritsky E, Hirshberg A. Maxillary sinus augmentation in the presence of antral pseudocyst: a clinical approach. Oral Surg Oral Med Oral Pathol Oral Radiol Endod 2007; 103: 180–184

[24] Cortes AR, Corrêa L, Arita ES. Evaluation of a maxillary sinus floor augmentation in the presence of a large antral pseudocyst. J Craniofac Surg 2012; 23: e535–e537

[25] Kara MI, Kirmali O, Ay S. Clinical evaluation of lateral and osteotome techniques for sinus floor elevation in the presence of an antral pseudocyst. Int J Oral Maxillofac Implants 2012; 27: 1205–1210

Index